Second Edition

# Companion Workbook for Human Histology

As per the latest NMC Guidelines | Competency Based Medical Education (CBME) Curriculum under Graduate Medical Education Regulation

**Ujwala Bhanarkar** MBBS MD
Assistant Professor
Department of Anatomy
All India Institute of Medical Sciences (AIIMS)
Kalyani, Kolkata, West Bengal, India

**Yogesh Ashok Sontakke** MBBS MD
Additional Professor
Department of Anatomy
Jawaharlal Institute of Postgraduate Medical Education and Research (JIPMER)
(An Institute of National Importance under the Ministry of Health and Family Welfare, Government of India)
Puducherry, India

CBSPD

**CBS Publishers & Distributors** Pvt Ltd

New Delhi • Bengaluru • Chennai • Kochi • Kolkata • Lucknow • Mumbai
Hyderabad • Jharkhand • Nagpur • Patna • Pune • Uttarakhand

# Contents


Plate 1: Parts of Microscope 3
Plate 2: Hematoxylin and Eosin Pencils 3
Plate 3: Structures Stained by Hematoxylin and Eosin 3
Plate 4: Cell and Cell Organelles 4
Plate 5: Microvilli, Stereocilia and Cilia 4
Plate 6: Simple Epithelium 4
Plate 7: Pseudostratified Columnar Epithelium 4
Plate 8: Non-keratinized Stratified Squamous 5
Plate 9: Keratinized Stratified Squamous 5
Plate 10: Transitional Epithelium 5
Plate 11: Serous Salivary Gland 6
Plate 12: Predominantly Mucous Salivary Gland 6
Plate 13: Mixed Salivary Gland 7
Plate 14: Types of Connective Tissue Fibers 7
Plate 15: Loose Connective (Areolar) Tissue 8
Plate 16: Dens Regular Connective Tissue (Tendon) 8
Plate 17: Yellow Adipose Tissue 9
Plate 18: Hyaline Cartilage 9
Plate 19: Elastic Cartilage 10
Plate 20: White Fibrocartilage 10
Plate 21: Transverse Section (TS) of Dry, Compact Bone 11
Plate 22: Longitudinal Section (LS) of Dry, Compact Bone 11
Plate 23: Cancellous (Trabecular or Spongy) Bone 12
Plate 24: Developing Bone 12
Plate 25: Skeletal Muscle 13
Plate 26: Cardiac Muscle 13
Plate 27: Smooth Muscles 14
Plate 28: Lymph Node 14
Plate 29: Spleen 15
Plate 30: Palatine Tonsil 15
Plate 31: Thymus 16
Plate 32: Peripheral Nerve—Transverse Section 16
Plate 33: Peripheral Myelinated Nerve—Osmic Acid Stanning 17
Plate 34: Dorsal Root or Spinal Ganglion 17
Plate 35: Autonomic or Sympathetic Ganglion 18
Plate 36: Large or Elastic Artery 18
Plate 37: Medium-sized or Muscular Artery 19
Plate 38: Arteriole and Venule 19
Plate 39: Types of Capillaries 20
Plate 40: Medium-sized Vein 20
Plate 41: Large Vein 21
Plate 42: Thin Skin 21
Plate 43: Thick Skin 22
Plate 44: Epiglottis 22
Plate 45: Trachea 23
Plate 46: Lung 23
Plate 47: Lip 24
Plate 48: Tooth 24
Plate 49: Tongue: Anterior Two-thirds 25
Plate 50: Types of Papillae 25
Plate 51: Tongue: Posterior One-third 26
Plate 52: Esophagus (Lower Part) 26
Plate 53: Gastro-esophageal Junction 27
Plate 54: Stomach: Fundus and Body 27
Plate 55: Stomach: Pylorus 28
Plate 56: Duodenum 28
Plate 57: Jejunum 29
Plate 58: Ileum 29
Plate 59: Large Intestine 30
Plate 60: Appendix 30
Plate 61: Liver 31
Plate 62: Gallbladder 31
Plate 63: Pancreas 32
Plate 64: Kidney 32
Plate 65: Ureter 33
Plate 66: Urinary Bladder 33
Plate 67: Testis 34
Plate 68: Epididymis 34
Plate 69: Ductus Deferens/Vas Deferens 35
Plate 70: Seminal Vesicle 35
Plate 71: Prostate 36
Plate 72: Penis 36
Plate 73: Ovary 37
Plate 74: Uterus: Proliferative Phase 37
Plate 75: Uterus: Secretory Phase 38
Plate 76: Cervix of Uterus 38
Plate 77: Fallopian Tube 39
Plate 78: Mammary Gland: Inactive Stage 39
Plate 79: Mammary Gland: In Lactation 40
Plate 80: Placenta 40
Plate 81: Umbilical Cord 41
Plate 82: Pituitary Gland 41
Plate 83: Suprarenal/Adrenal Gland 42
Plate 84: Thyroid Gland 42
Plate 85: Parathyroid Gland 43
Plate 86: Cerebrum 43
Plate 87: Cerebellum 44
Plate 88: Spinal Cord (H&E Staining) 44
Plate 89: Spinal Cord at Different Levels 45
Plate 90: Cornea 45
Plate 91: Retina 46
Plate 92: Optic Nerve—Transverse Section 46
Plate 93: Cochlea 47

# Preface

In the practical histology laboratory, learning to identify histological structures is an expected learning outcome. The identification of the histological structure should be supported with specific points. As per the latest CBME curriculum and GMER-2019, a separate weightage is given to the logbooks. This practical companion book is prepared with the intention of providing a guide to students to draw easy and beautiful diagrams in their logbooks. It will also help in preparation for Histology practical examination and viva.

**Ujwala Bhanarkar**
**Yogesh Ashok Sontakke**

## HISTOLOGY DIAGRAMS

### Plate 1: Parts of Microscope

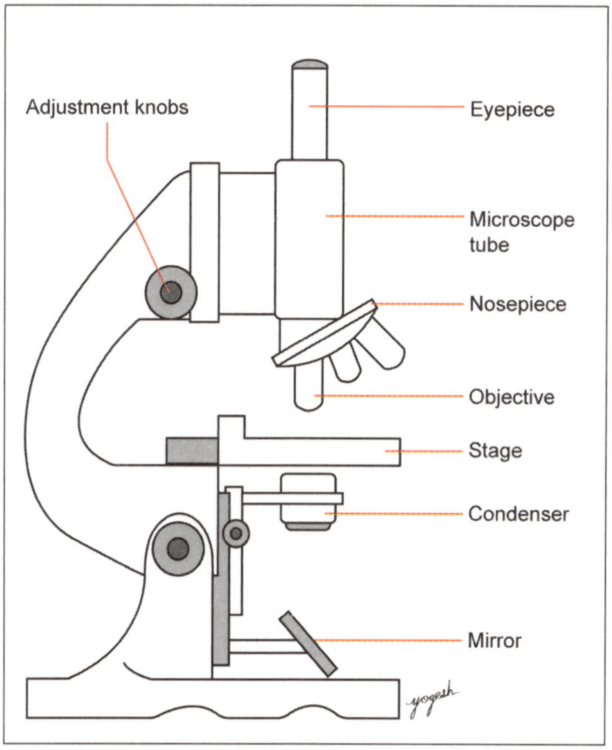


*Note*: Draw this figure using Hb pencil.

### Plate 2: Hematoxylin and Eosin Pencils

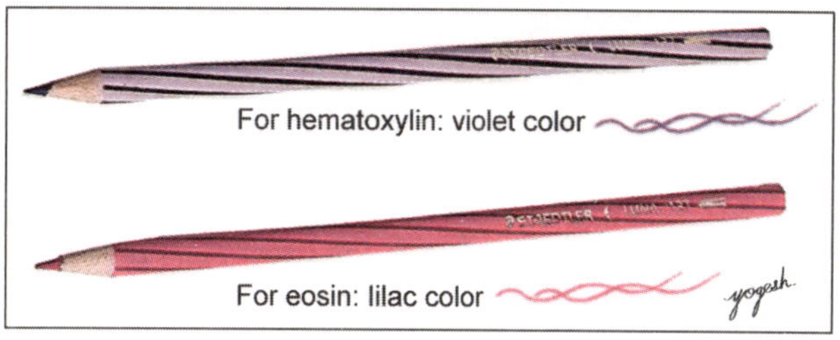


### Plate 3: Structures Stained by Hematoxylin and Eosin

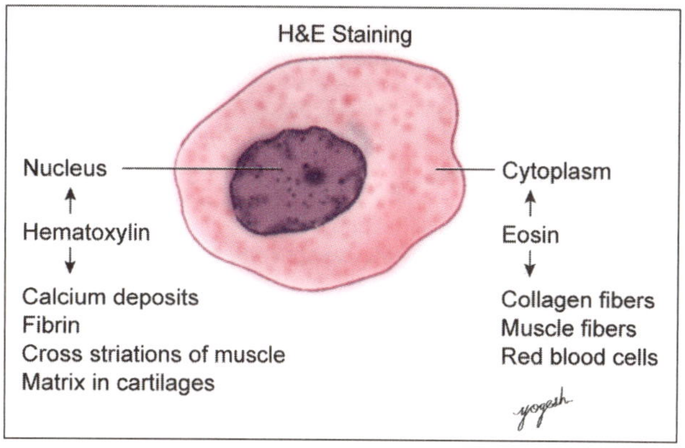


- For drawing diagrams, always use special violet and lilac color professional pencils for drawing hematoxylin and eosin-stained structures (Apsara, Faber-Castell, Staedtler or any other suitable brand). Do not use routine pink and violet color pencils. Use HB pencil or black pen for labeling.
- Hematoxylin stains nuclei, calcium deposits, fibrin, cross striations of muscle, matrix in cartilages, and so on. Eosin is an acidic type that stains basic or eosinophilic compounds such as cytoplasm, connective tissue (collagen fibers), muscle fibers, red blood cells, and so on.

*Space for Notes* ____

## Plate 4: Cell and Cell Organelles

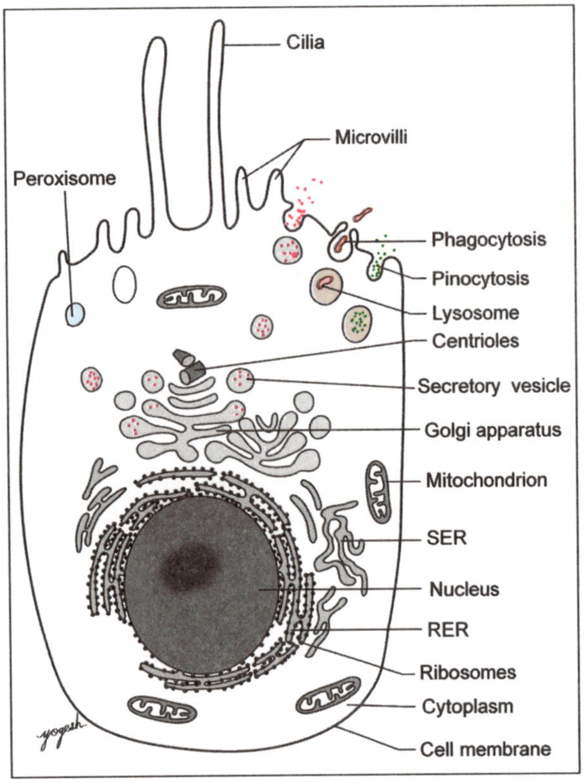


(RER: Rough endoplasmic reticulum, SER: Smooth endoplasmic reticulum, draw this diagram using HB pencil)

## Plate 5: Microvilli, Stereocilia and Cilia

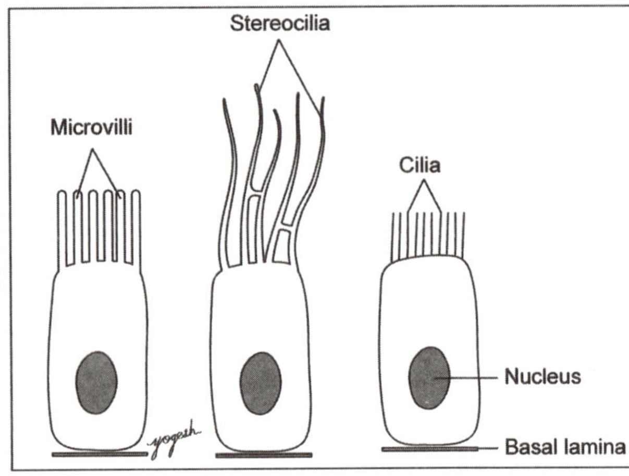


- Microvilli are apical cell surface modifications that increase cell surface area for absorption or secretion.
- Stereocilia is a long, thick, nonmotile microvillus (5–10 μm).
- Cilia are apical cell membranous hair-like motile projections (~10 μm).

## Plate 6: Simple Epithelium

***Simple squamous epithelium***

Single layer of flat cells
Oval or flat nucleus
***Locations***: Endothelium, lung alveoli, parietal layers of Bowman's capsule

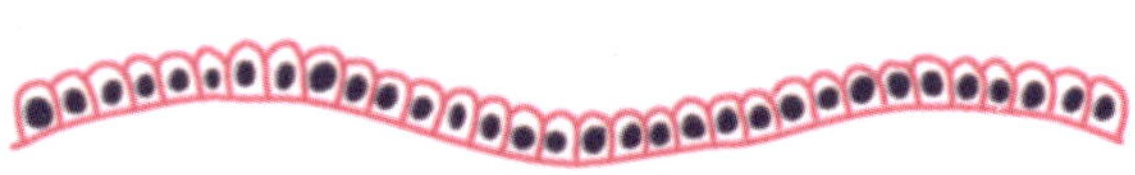

***Simple cuboid epithelium***

Single layer of cuboidal cells
Rounded, centrally placed nucleus
***Locations***: Thyroid follicles, small duct of glands, DCT in kidney

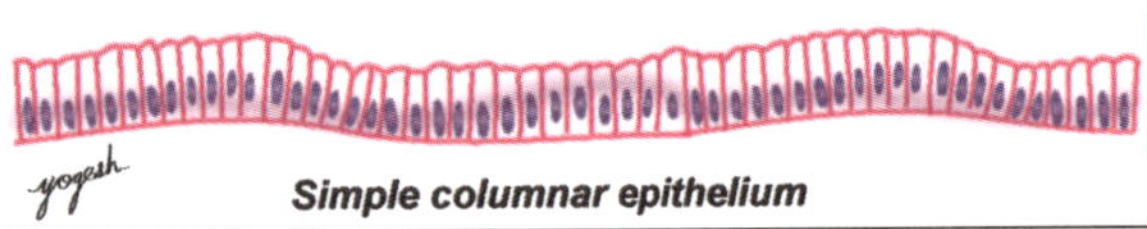

***Simple columnar epithelium***

Single layer of columnar cells
Oval (elongated), basally located nuclei
***Locations***: Intestine, stomach, gallbladder, uterus, fallopian tube

*Note*: Draw each of these diagrams in a separate circle.

## Plate 7: Pseudostratified Columnar Epithelium

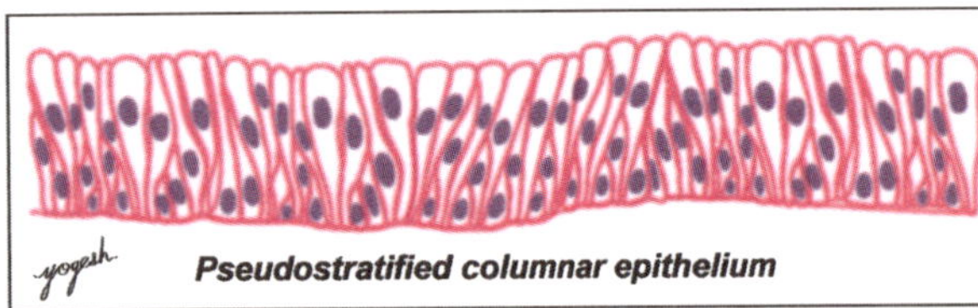

***Pseudostratified columnar epithelium***

Simple epithelium, false impression of stratification
All cells attached to basement membrane
Cells have different heights
***Locations***: Respiratory epithelium (ciliated); noncilated in auditory tube, ductus deferens, part of male urethra

*Space for Notes* ____________________

## Plate 8: **Nonkeratinized Stratified Squamous Epithelium**

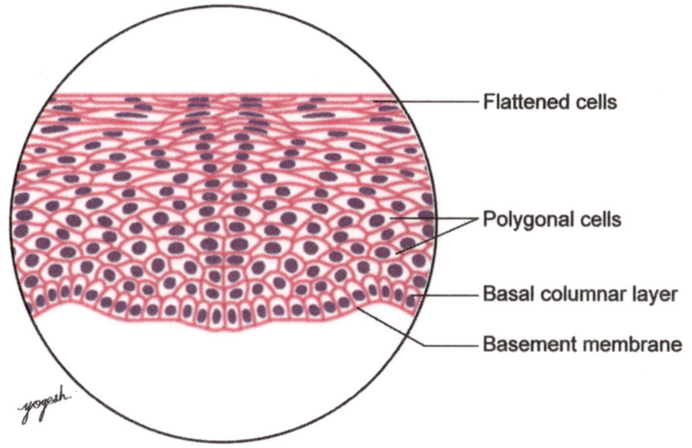


Multiple layers of cells
Cells of uppermost layer are nucleated (no stratum corneum)
***Locations***: Oral cavity, oropharynx, esophagus, vagina, cornea

## Plate 9: **Keratinized Squamous Epithelium**

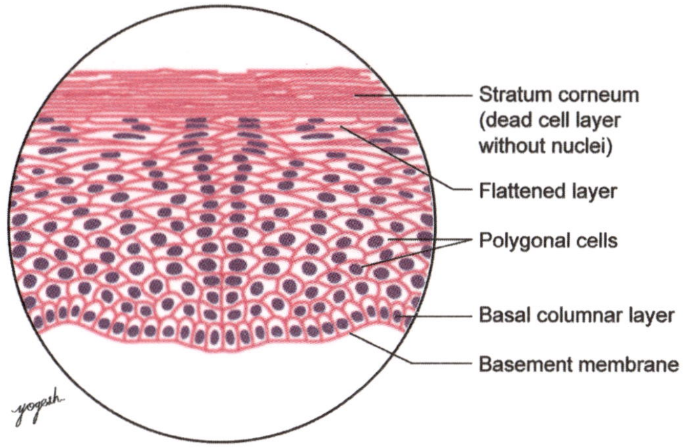


Multiple layers of cells
Superficial dead cell layer—called stratum corneum
***Location***: Epidermis of skin

## Plate 10: **Transitional Epithelium (Urothelium)**

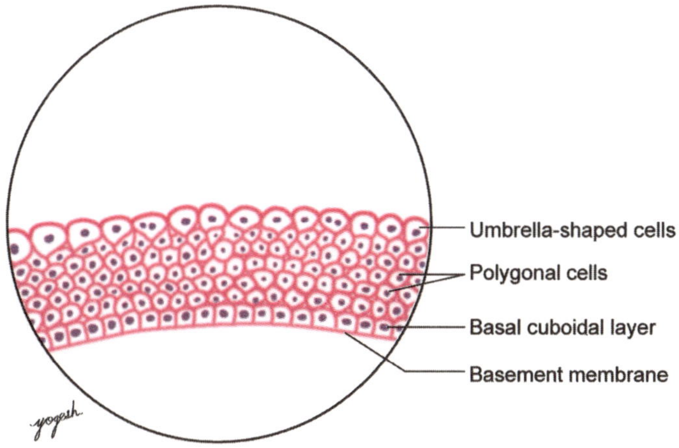


3–5 cell-layer thick
Basal cuboidal cells
Intermediate polygonal cells
Superficial umbrella (dome)-shaped cells (may be binucleated)—more eosinophilic due to plaques of glycoproteins
***Location***: Urinary bladder, ureter

*Space for Notes* ________________________________

## Plate 11: Serous Salivary Gland

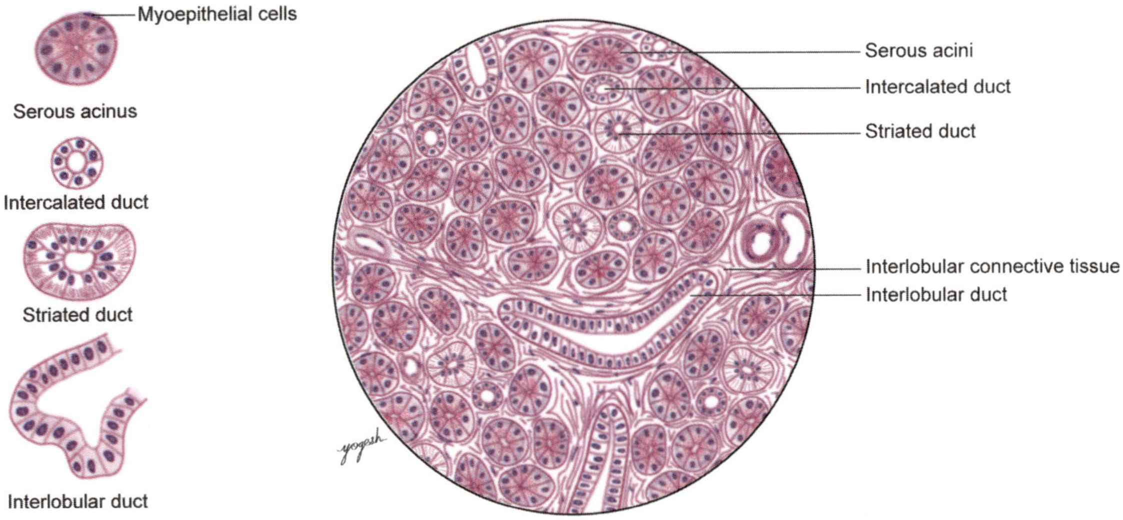


Serous acinus: Smaller than mucous acini with narrow lumen
Lined by simple columnar epithelium with round and basally placed nuclei
Cytoplasm: Basal basophlia and apical eosinophilia
Ducts: Intercalated ducts lined by cuboidal epithelium
Striated ducts lined by columnar epithelium with basal infoldings of cell membrane
Interlobular ducts lined by columnar cells

***Example***
Parotid gland

## Plate 12: Predominantly Mucous Salivary Gland (Sublingual Salivary Gland)

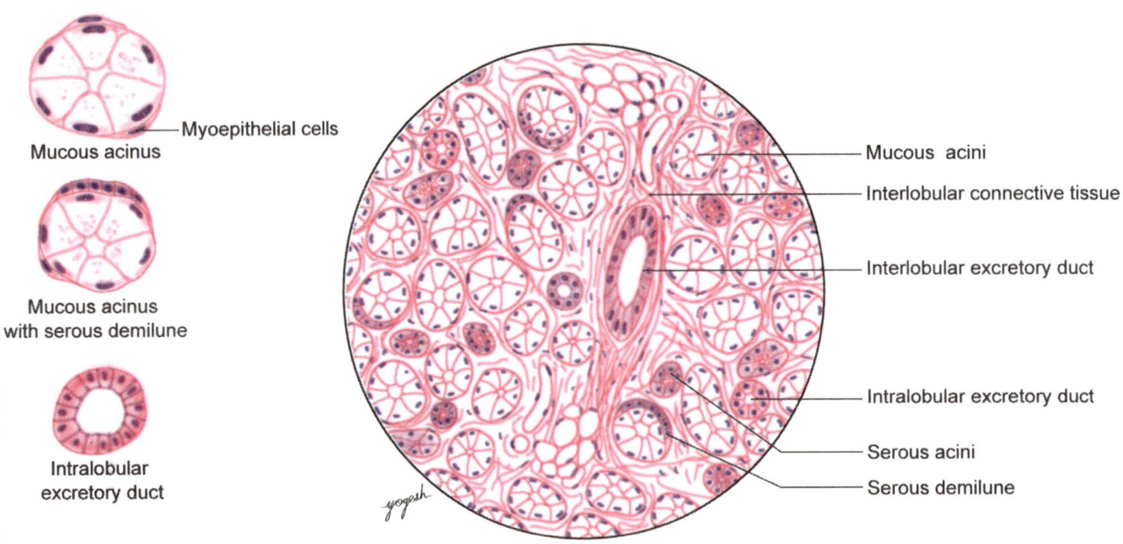


Predominantly mucous acini are present
Mucous acinus: Larger than serous acini with larger lumen
Lined by simple columnar epithelium with flat, elongated and basally placed nucleus
Foamy cytoplasm (mucus removed during tissue processing)
Intralobular ducts lined by cuboidal epithelium and interlobular ducts lined by columnar cells

***Example***
Sublingual salivary gland

*Space for Notes*

## Plate 13: **Mixed Salivary Gland (Submandibular Gland)**

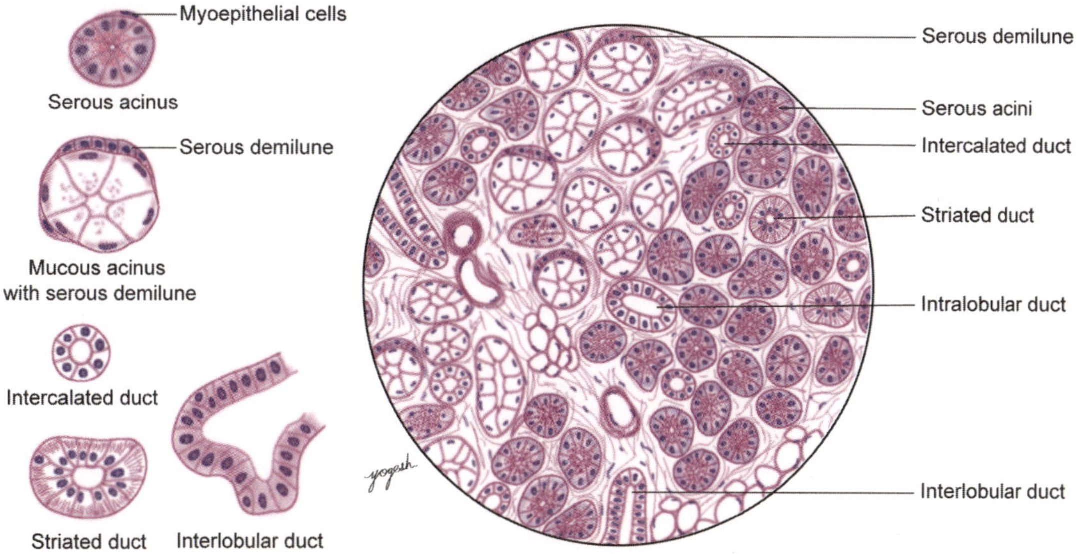


Acini: Smaller serous acini with narrow lumen
Mucous acini with wider lumen
Serous demilunes cap the mucous acini

Ducts: Intercalated ducts lined by cuboidal epithelium
Striated ducts lined by columnar epithelium with basal infoldings of cell membrane
Interlobular ducts lined by columnar cells

***Example***
Submandibular salivary gland

## Plate 14: **Connective Tissue Fibers**

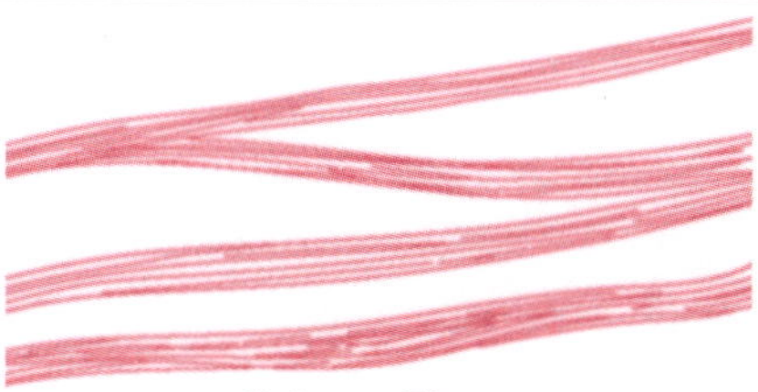

Collagen Fibers

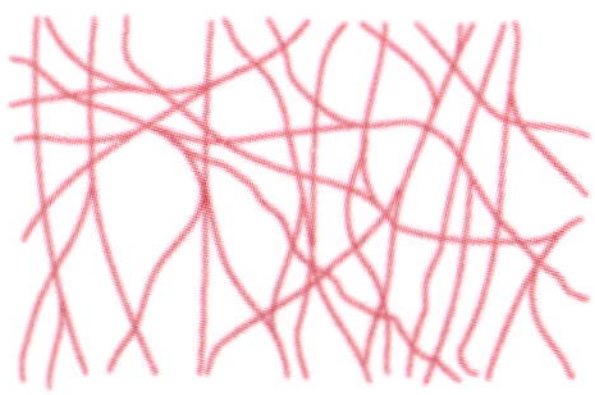

Elastic Fibers

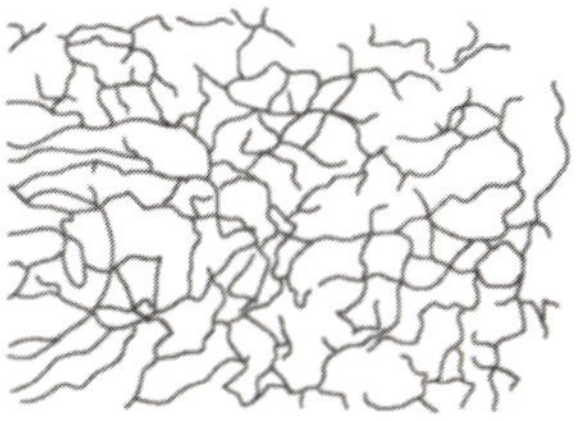

Reticular Fibers

Most abundant fibers
Runs in bundles, Bundles are branching
Location: Tendons, ligaments

Runs singly and branch
Location: Large vessels, lungs
Special stain: Orcein, Verhoeff's

Form mesh-like network
Location: Liver, spleen, lymph nodes
Special stain: Silver impregnation

*Space for Notes* ____________________

## Plate 15: **Loose (Areolar) Connective Tissue**

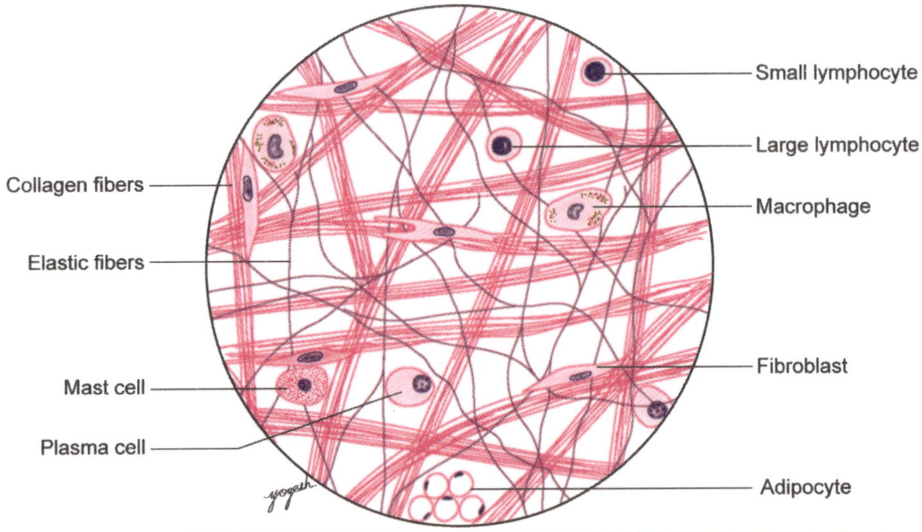


It consists of cells, fibers, and extracellular matrix.
Cells are resident cells (fibroblasts, adipocytes, etc.) and wandering cells (lymphocytes, plasma cells, etc.).
Connective tissue fibers consist of collagen, elastic, and reticular fibers.
Extracellular matrix is a supportive amorphous substance that consists of proteoglycans, glycoproteins, and glycosaminoglycans.
Location: Mesentery, lamina propria, superficial fascia

## Plate 16: **Dense Regular Connective Tissue (Longitudinal Section of Tendon)**

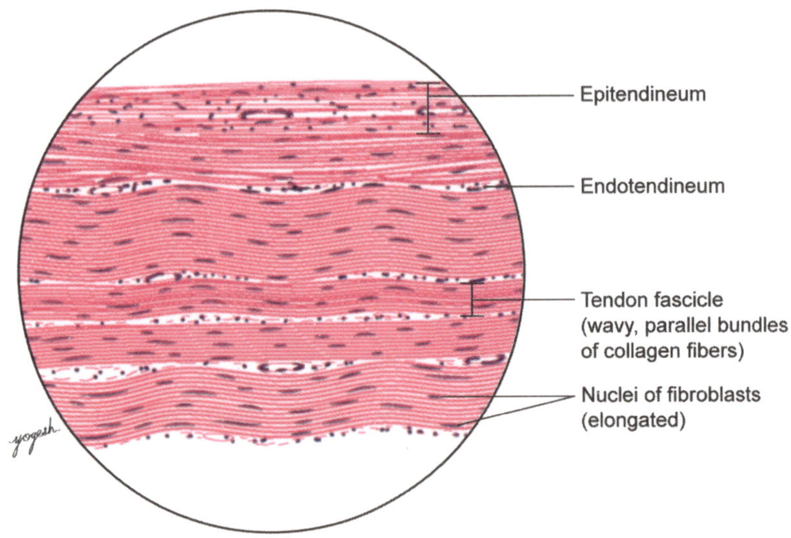


Collagen fibers are arranged in compact parallel array of thick bundles (cord pattern).
Bundles of collagen fibers show wavy appearance.
Fibroblasts (tendinocytes) are elongated cells, oriented along the long axis of collagen bundles.
Endotendineum is vascular connective tissue layer that separates the bundles.
Epitendineum covers entire tendon.

***Examples***
Tendon, ligament

*Space for Notes* ____________________

## Plate 17: **Yellow Adipose Tissue**

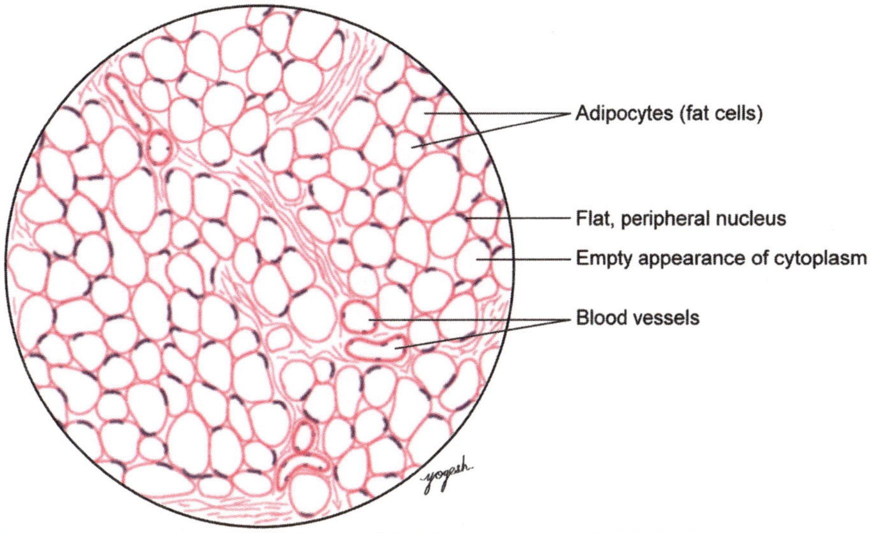


Adipocytes are large oval cells with flat peripheral nuclei and very thin rims of cytoplasm (signet ring appearance)
As fat gets washed out during tissue processing, cells appear empty
Locations: Superficial fascia (breast, buttocks), yellow bone marrow

## Plate 18: **Hyaline Cartilage**

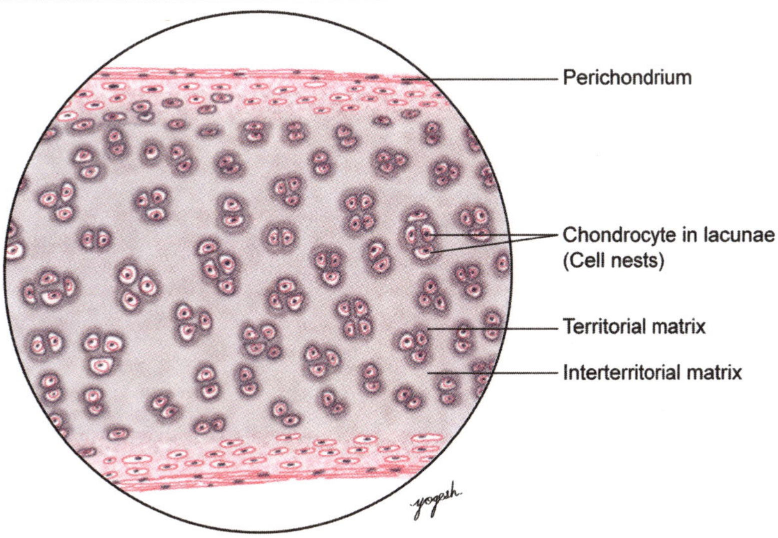


- Chondrocytes are present in isogenous group of 2–6 cells or cell nests.
- Homogeneous (amorphous) basophilic matrix (ground-glass appearance)
- Perichondrium surrounds the cartilage
- Locations: Nasal septum, tracheal rings, costal cartilages

*Space for Notes* ________

## Plate 19: **Elastic Cartilage**

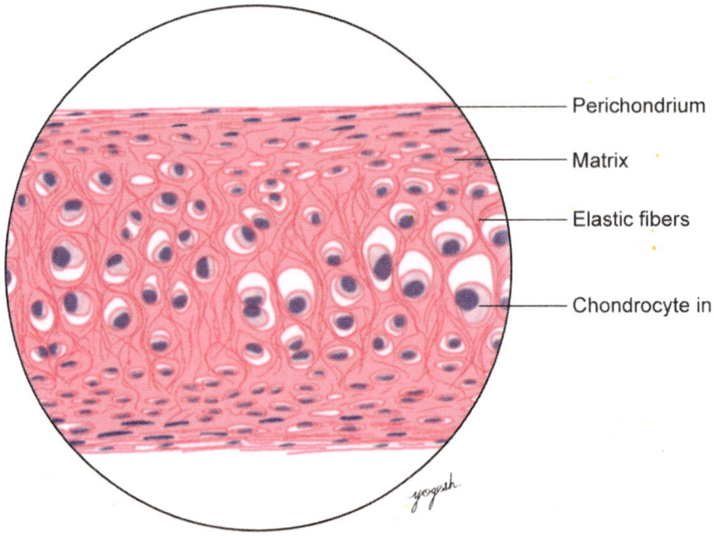


- Large and few chondrocytes lie singly or in groups of two
- Matrix shows eosinophilic branching fibers
- Perichondrium surrounds cartilage
- Locations: Pinna of external ear, epiglottis, auditory tube

## Plate 20: **White Fibrocartilage**

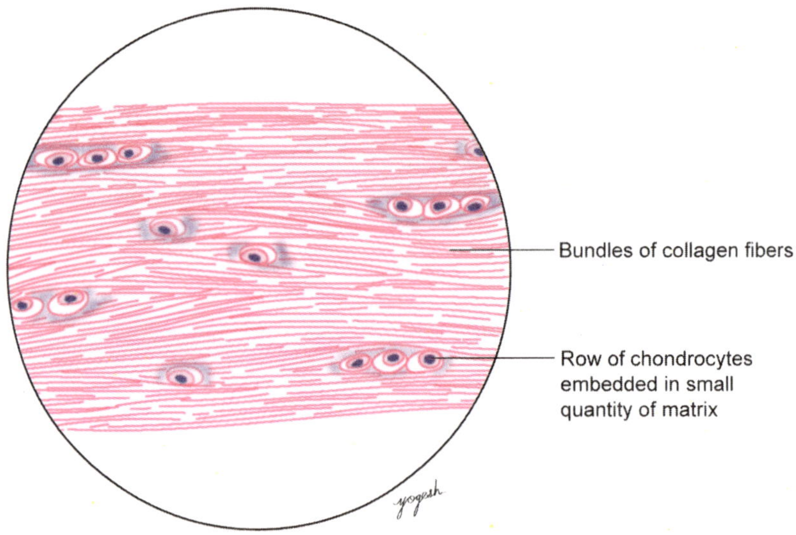


Consists of bundles of collagen fibers with interspaced rows of few small chondrocytes
Perichondrium is absent
Locations: Intervertebral discs, menisci of knee joint, pubic symphysis

*Space for Notes* __________

## Plate 21: **Transverse Section (TS) of Dry, Compact Bone**

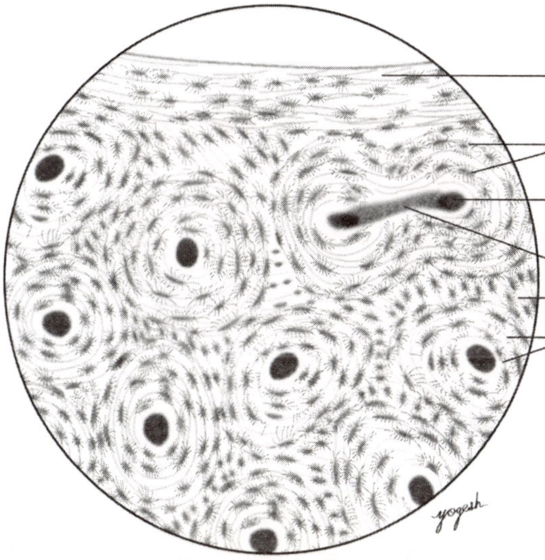


Osteons has central Haversian canal surrounded by concentric lamellae
Lacunae are present in between adjacent lamellae
Osteocytes lie in lacunae
Volkman's canals connect adjacent Haversian canals
Interstitial and outer and inner circumferential lamellae are present

## Plate 22: **Longitudinal Section (LS) of Dry, Compact Bone**

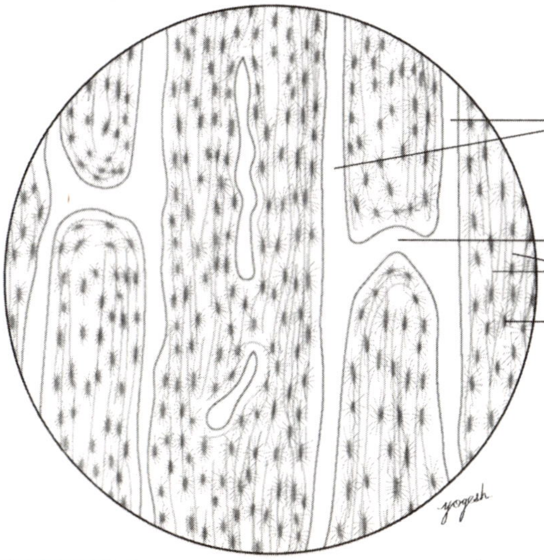


Longitudinally running Haversian canals are present which are connected in horizontal Volkmann's canals
Lamellae and lacunae surround the canals
Lacunae contains osteocytes

*Space for Notes*

## Plate 23: Cancellous (Trabecular or Spongy) Bone

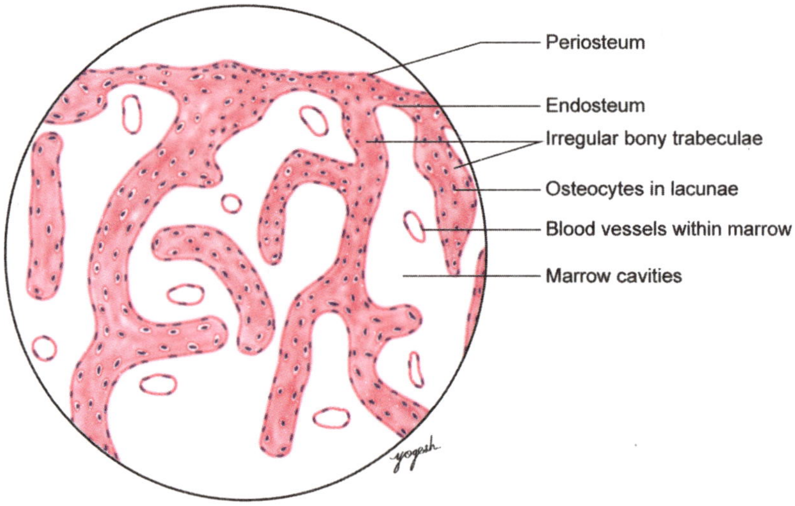


Meshwork of irregularly arranged trabeculae that encloses spaces called bone marrow.
Trabeculae contains lacunae with osteocytes and lamellae
No Haversian system.

## Plate 24: Developing Bone

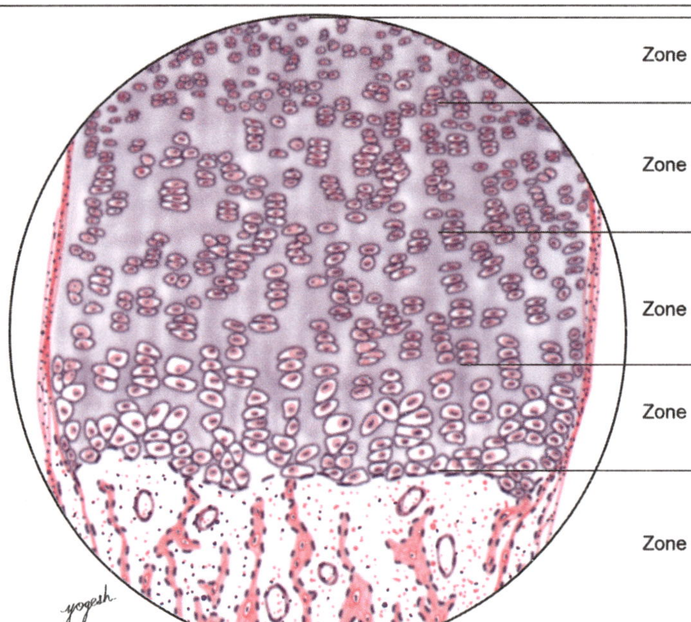


5 zones:
1. Zone of reserve cartilage: Small, singly lying chrondrocytes
2. Zone of proliferation: Larger and numerous chondrocytes
3. Zone of hypertrophy: Bigger chrondrocytes arranged in columns.
4. Zone of calcified cartilage: Calcium in extracellular matrix with dying chondrocytes.
5. Zone of resorption: Longitudinal bony spicules with osteoblasts.

Location:
Epiphyseal cartilage

*Space for Notes*

## Plate 25: **Skeletal Muscle**

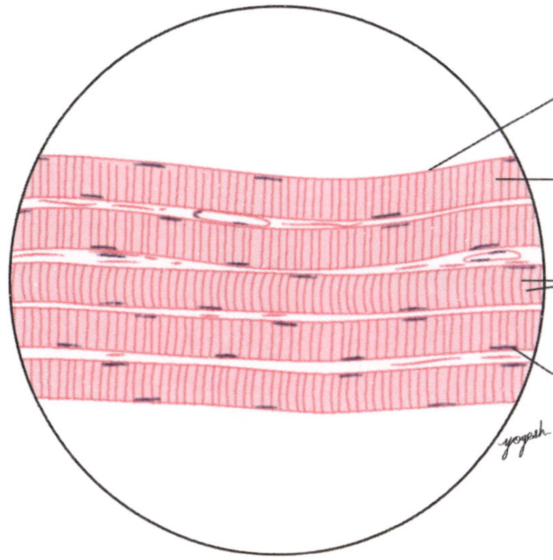


Multinucleated, long, parallel, nonbranching muscle fibers
Multiple, flat, peripheral nuclei
Alterate dark and light bands (striations)

## Plate 26: **Cardiac Muscle**

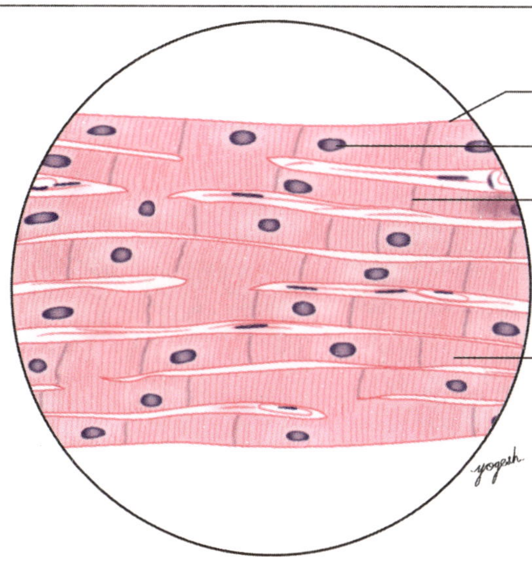


Single nucleated, short branching muscle fibers
Single, oval central nucleus with perinuclear halo
Less prominent alternate dark and light bands (striations)
Darkly-strained intercalated discs

*Space for Notes* ____________________

## Plate 27: **Smooth Muscles**

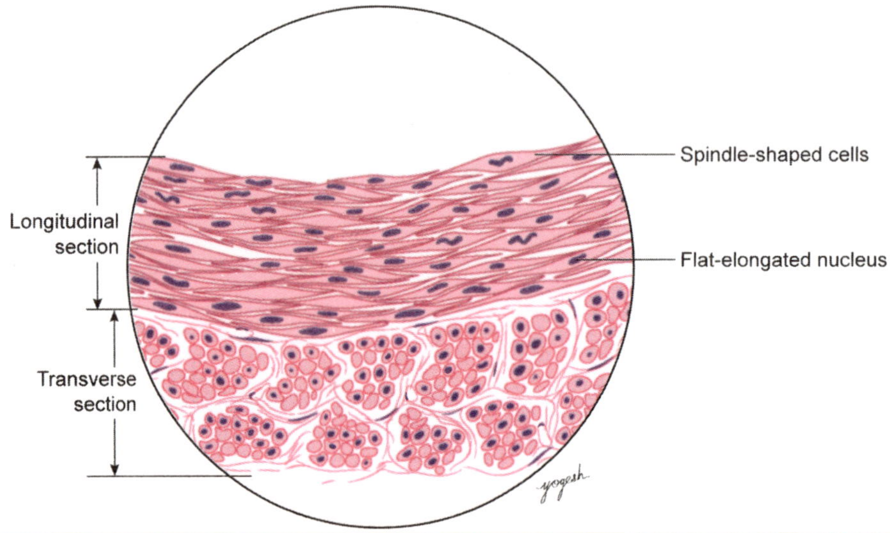


Small, spindle-shaped muscle cells
Central elongated nucleus
Striations are absent
In longitudinal section: Cells are circular with central round nuclei
Location: Wall of intestine, wall of ureter

## Plate 28: **Lymph Node**

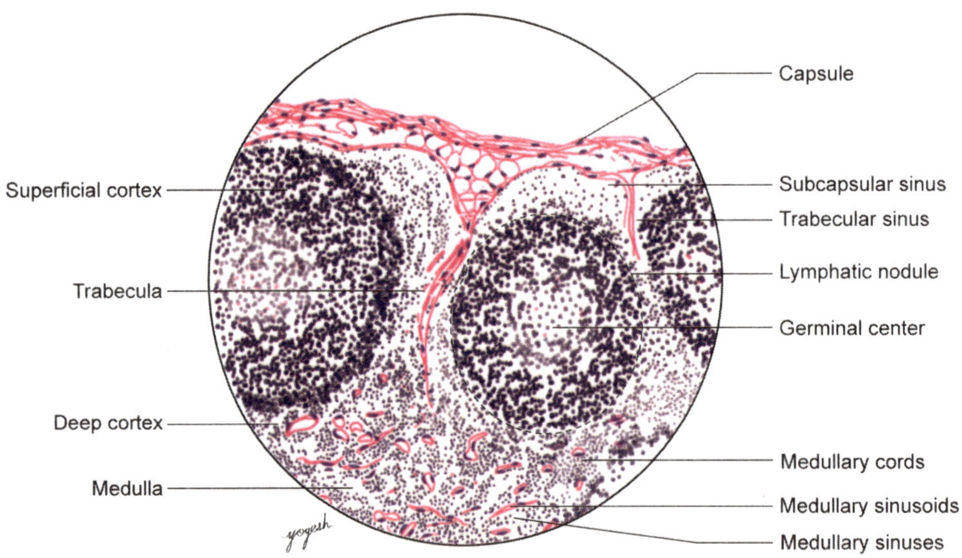


Lymph node has connective tissue capsule, outer darkly stained superficial and deep cortices, and inner lightly stained medulla.
Cortex shows lymphatic nodules, and medulla consists of cords of B lymphocytes separated by anastomosing medullary sinuses.
Subcapsular sinus lies beneath the capsule, trabecular sinuses connect subcapsular sinus with medullary sinuses
Functions: Filtration of lymph, presentation of antigens to T cells, production of antibodies

*Space for Notes* __________

## Plate 29: **Spleen**

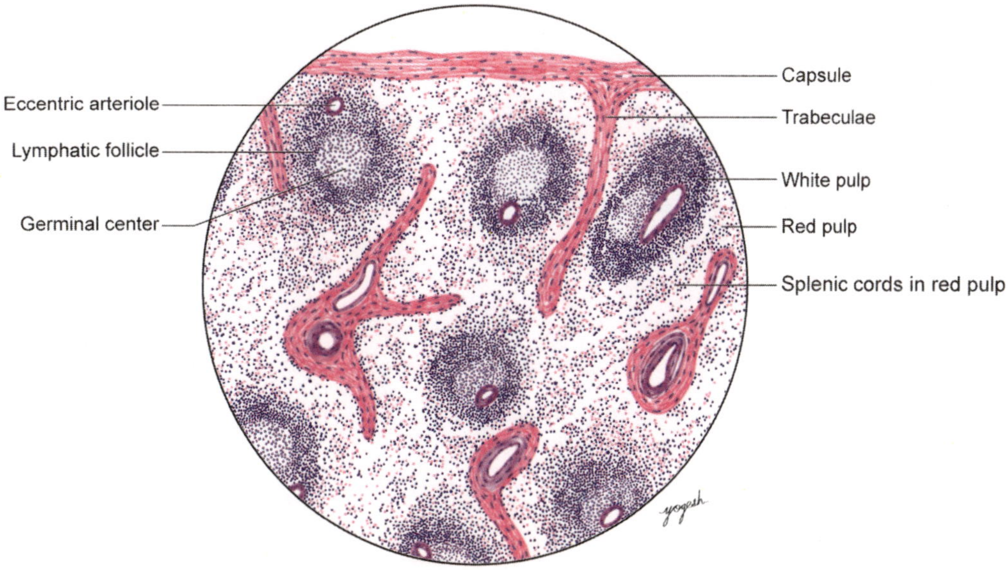


Spleen is covered by thick capsule that sends trabeculae into the parenchyma of spleen.
Spleen shows:
White pulp—consists of splenic nodules/Malpighian corpuscles with germinal center and eccentric arterioles
Red pulp—consists of diffuse cords of Billroth (made up of RBCs, lymphocytes, macrophages, and plasma cells)
Functions: Immune functions (activates lymphocytes and induces immune response), destruction of old and damaged RBCs and platelets.

## Plate 30: **Platine Tonsil**

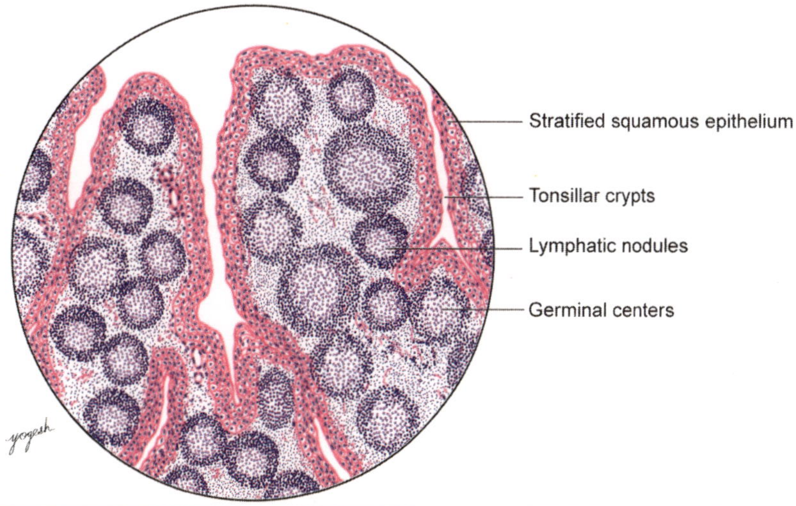


Palatine tonsil shows lining epithelium, tonsillar crypts, lymphatic follicles, and connective tissue capsule.
Oral surface of the palatine tonsil is covered by nonkeratinized stratified squamous epithelium, which invaginates to form tonsillar crypts.
Just beneath epithelium, dense aggregation of lymphatic follicles is present.
Functions: Production of lymphocytes, antigen presentation, and development of immune response.

*Space for Notes* ______

## Plate 31: **Thymus**

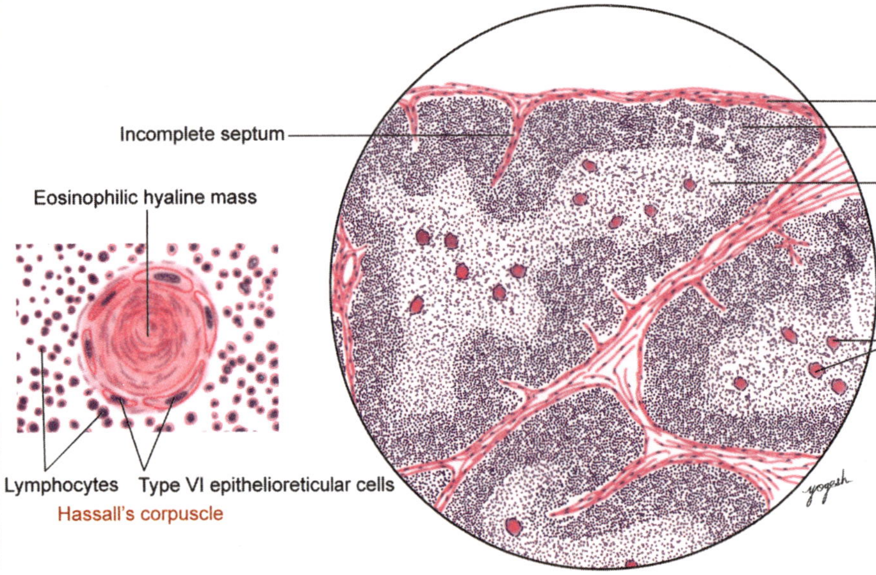


Thymus shows connective tissue capsule and incomplete septa that divide thymus into number of incomplete lobules.
It has outer darkly stained cortex and inner lightly stained medulla.
Medulla of adjacent lobules is continuous with each other.
Medulla shows *Hassall's corpuscles*—a central pink hyalinized material surrounded by type VI epithelioreticular cells.
Function: Production of mature T lymphocytes, secretion of thymosin and thymopoietin.

## Plate 32: **Peripheral Nerve — Transverse Section (H&E Staining)**

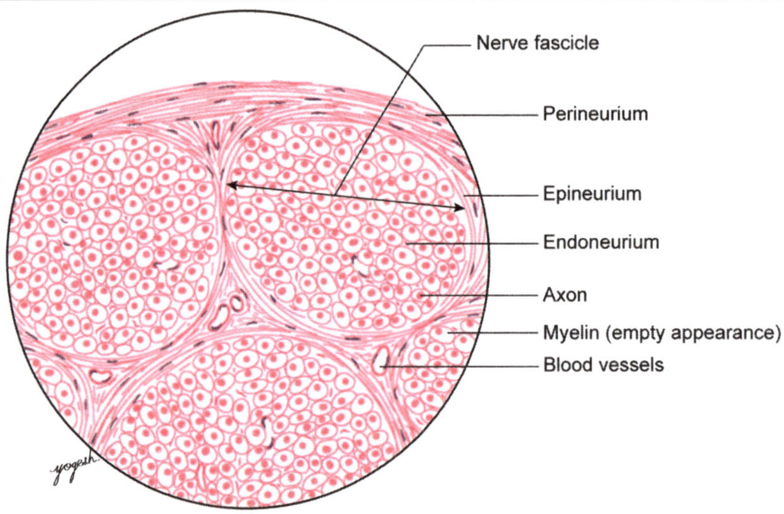


Each peripheral nerve consists of:
- Nerve fibers: Axons are surrounded by myelin (empty spaces) and endoneurium.
- Connective tissue coats:
  - Endoneurium—surrounds a single nerve fiber
  - Perineurium—surrounds nerve fascicles
  - Epineurium—surrounds bundles of nerve fascicles and entire nerve

*Space for Notes*

## Plate 33: **Peripheral Nerve – Osmic Acid Stain**

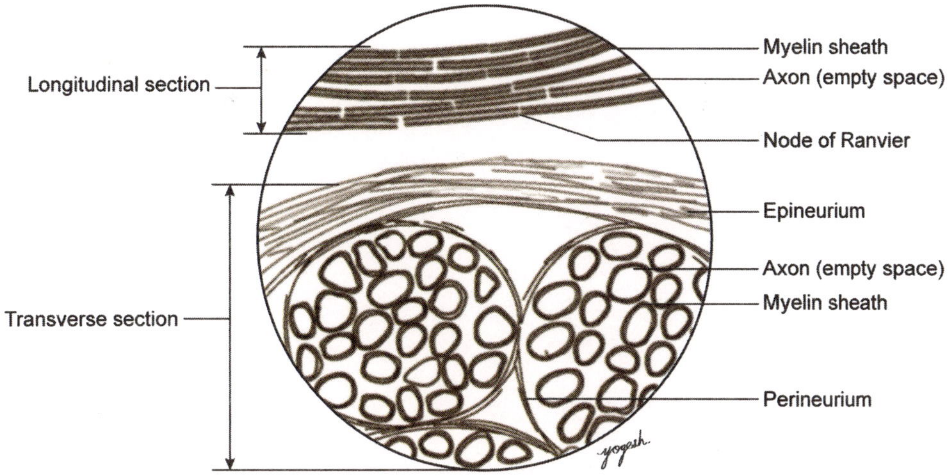


Peripheral nerve on osmic acid stain shows:

In longitudinal section: Thick, black bands of myelin sheaths around unstained axons.

The nodes of Ranvier are represented by gaps in myelin sheaths.

In transverse section: Thick, black rings of various diameters around unstained axons.

## Plate 34: **Dorsal Root Ganglion/Spinal Ganglion**

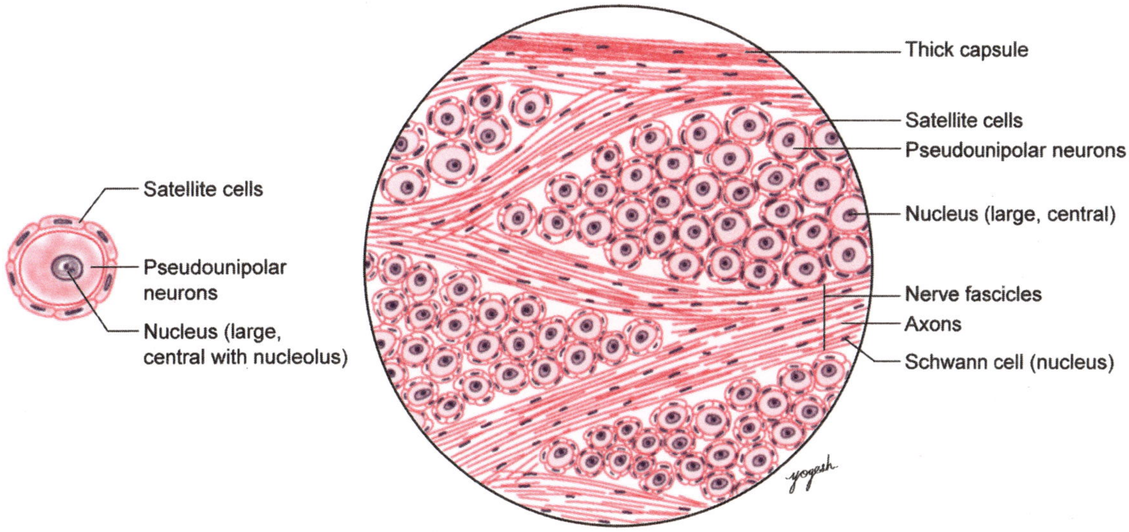


Pseudounipolar neuronal bodies are arranged in clusters (groups).

These neurons are large, spherical in shape with large, vesicular, and centrally placed nuclei.

Bundles of nerve fibers (myelinated) separate groups of neurons.

Satellite cells are flattened satellite cells form a complete ring around body of each neuron.

*Space for Notes* ____________________

## Plate 35: **Autonomic or Sympathetic Ganglion**

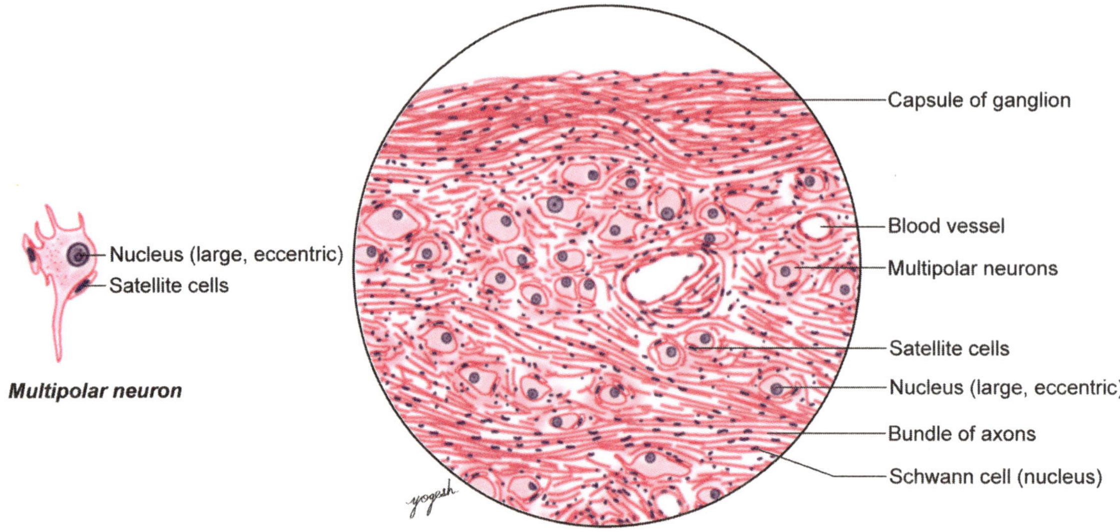


***Multipolar neuron***

Multipolar neurons are scattered among nerve fibers.
These neurons are large, irregular shaped with large, vesicular, and eccentrically placed nuclei.
Nerve fibers are arranged in bundles that run between scattered neurons.
Few flat satellite cells surround each nerve cell body but do not form a complete ring.

## Plate 36: **Large or Elastic Artery**

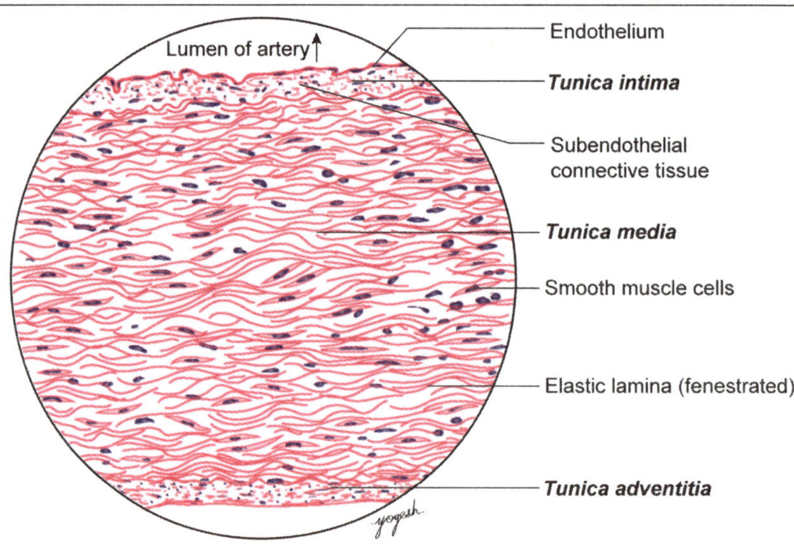


Elastic (large/conducting) artery consists of tunica intima, tunica media, and tunica adventitia.
Tunica intima shows endothelium (simple squamous epithelium), subendothelial connective tissue and indistinguishable internal elastic lamella.
Tunica media shows many layers of spindle-shaped vascular smooth muscle fibers and many thick sheets of fenestrated elastic lamellae.
Tunica adventitia is relatively thin connective tissue layer.

Examples:
Aorta, brachiocephalic, common carotid and subclavian arteries, pulmonary trunk

*Space for Notes* ____

## Plate 37: **Medium-sized or Muscular Artery**

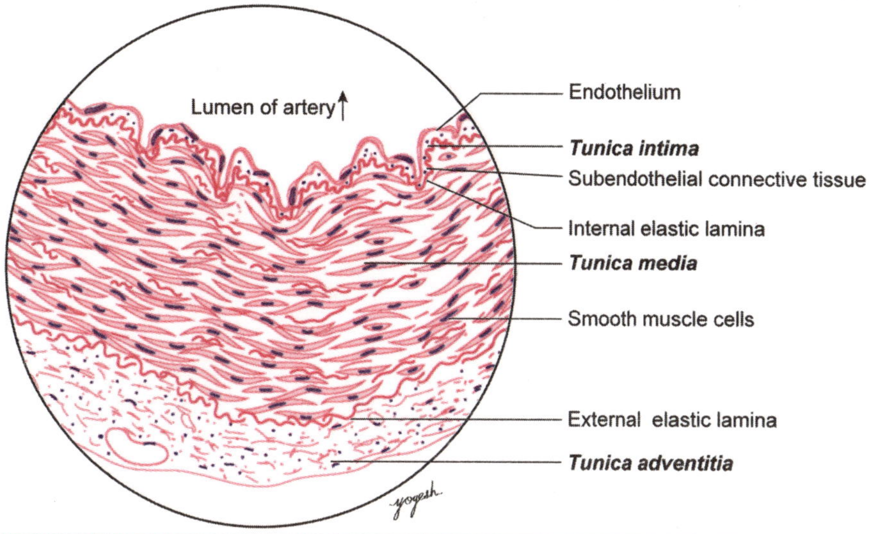


Muscular (medium-sized/distributing) artery consists of tunica intima, tunica media, and tunica adventitia.
Tunica intima = Endothelium (simple squamous epithelium) + scanty subendothelial connective tissue + prominent internal elastic lamina
Tunica media = layers of smooth muscle cells + few elastic fibers
Thick tunica adventitia

Examples:
Brachial artery, femoral artery

## Plate 38: **Arteriole and Venule**

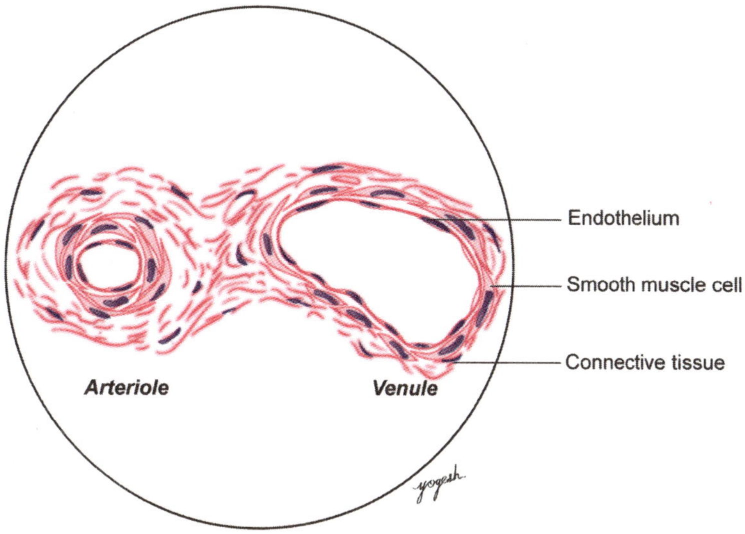


Arteriole consists of tunica intima (endothelium), tunica media (1–3 cell layers of smooth muscles), and tunica adventitia, thin tunica adventitia. Internal elastic lamina is mostly absent.
Venules are thinner than associated arterioles. They are lined by endothelium, 1–2 layers of smooth muscles and thick layer of connective tissue.

*Space for Notes*

## Plate 39: **Types of Capillaries**

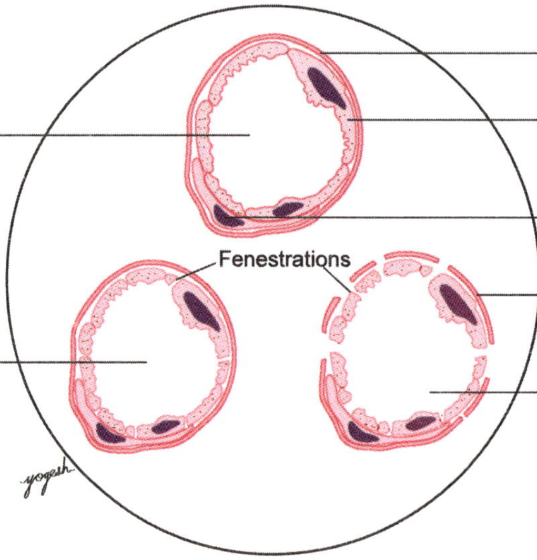


Continuous (somatic) capillaries have (uninterrupted vascular endothelium) and continuous basal lamina.
Fenestrated capillaries have endothelial cells with numerous circular openings (fenestrations) and continuous basal lamina.
Discontinuous or sinusoidal capillaries have endothelial cells with large pores or slits and discontinuous basal lamina.

## Plate 40: **Medium-sized Vein**

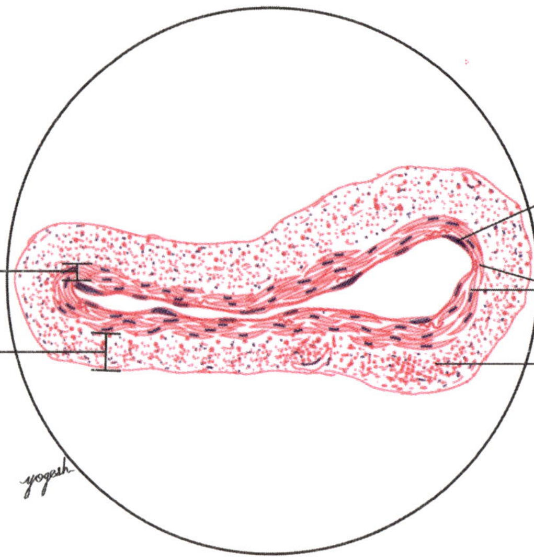


Medium-sized veins has poorly identifiable three layers tunica intima, tunica media, and tunica adventitia.
Tunica intima consists of endothelium, basal lamina, thin subendothelial connective tissue, and discontinuous internal elastic lamina.
Tunica media is thin and consists of few layers of smooth muscle cells.
Tunica adventitia is the thickest layer and has connective tissue.

Examples:
Radial vein, tibial vein, popliteal vein

*Space for Notes*

## Plate 41: **Large Vein**

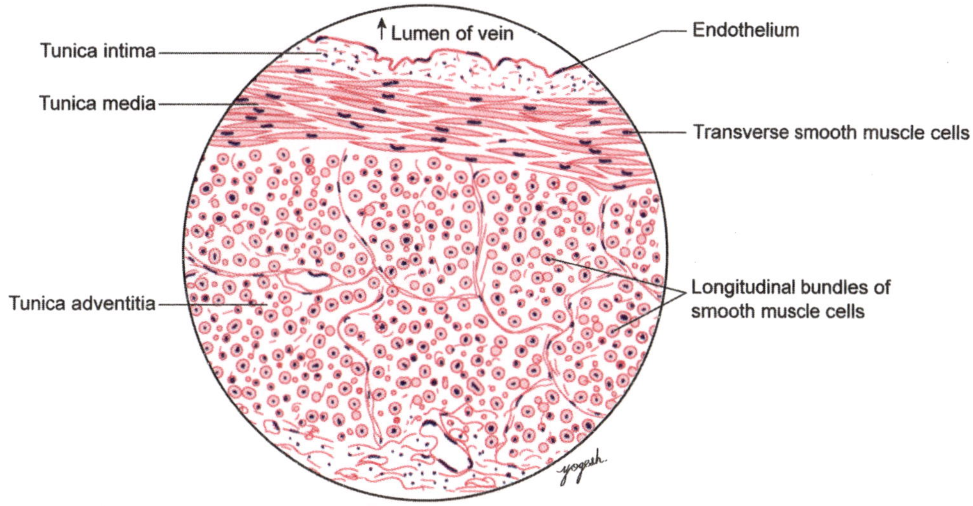


Large vein has three layers: Tunica intima, tunica media, and tunica adventitia.
Tunica intima has endothelium, basal lamina, and thin subendothelial connective tissue.
Tunica media has concentrically arranged smooth muscle cells, collagen fibers, and fibroblasts.
Tunica adventitia is the thickest layer and consists of longitudinally arranged smooth muscle cells.

***Examples***
Superior vena cava, interior vena cava.

## Plate 42: **Thin Skin**

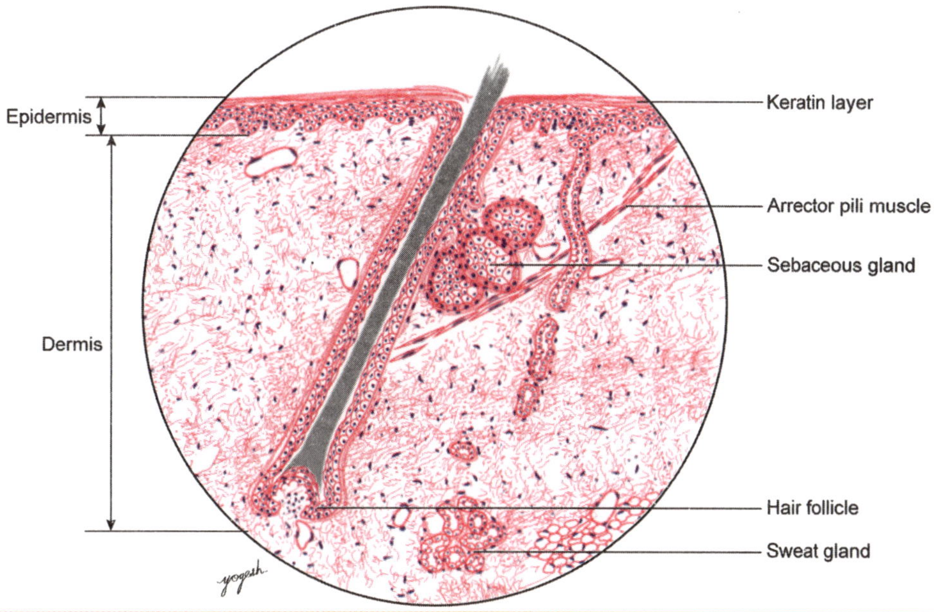


Skin has two layers: Superficial epidermis and deep dermis.
Outer epidermis is lined by keratinized stratified squamous epithelium
Inner dermis has connective tissue, *hair follicles*, sebaceous glands, arrector pili muscles, and sweat glands.
In thin skin, epidermis shows stratum basale (single layer of low columnar cells), stratum spinosum (several layers of polygonal cells), stratum granulosum (flattened cells), and stratum corneum (flat and dead cells).

*Space for Notes* ________________

## Plate 43: **Thick Skin**

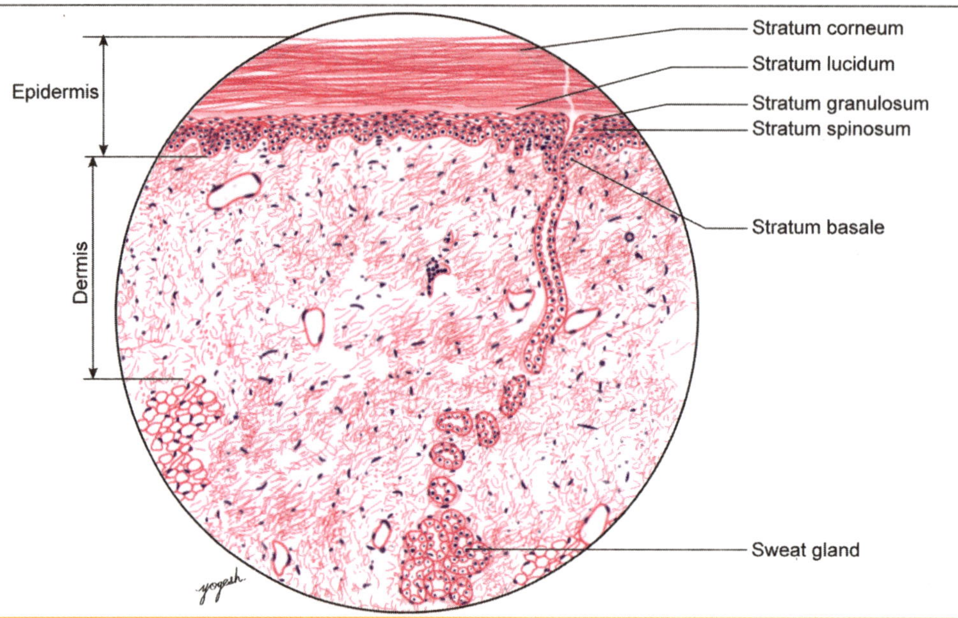


Skin has two layers: Superficial epidermis and deep dermis.
Outer epidermis is lined by keratinized stratified squamous epithelium
Inner dermis has connective tissue and sweat glands.
In thick skin, epidermis shows stratum basale (single layer of low columnar cells), stratum spinosum (several layers of polygonal cells), stratum granulosum (flattened cells), ***stratum lucidum*** (translucent layer), and ***thick stratum corneum*** (flat and dead cells).

Examples:
Skin of palm and sole

## Plate 44: **Epiglottis**

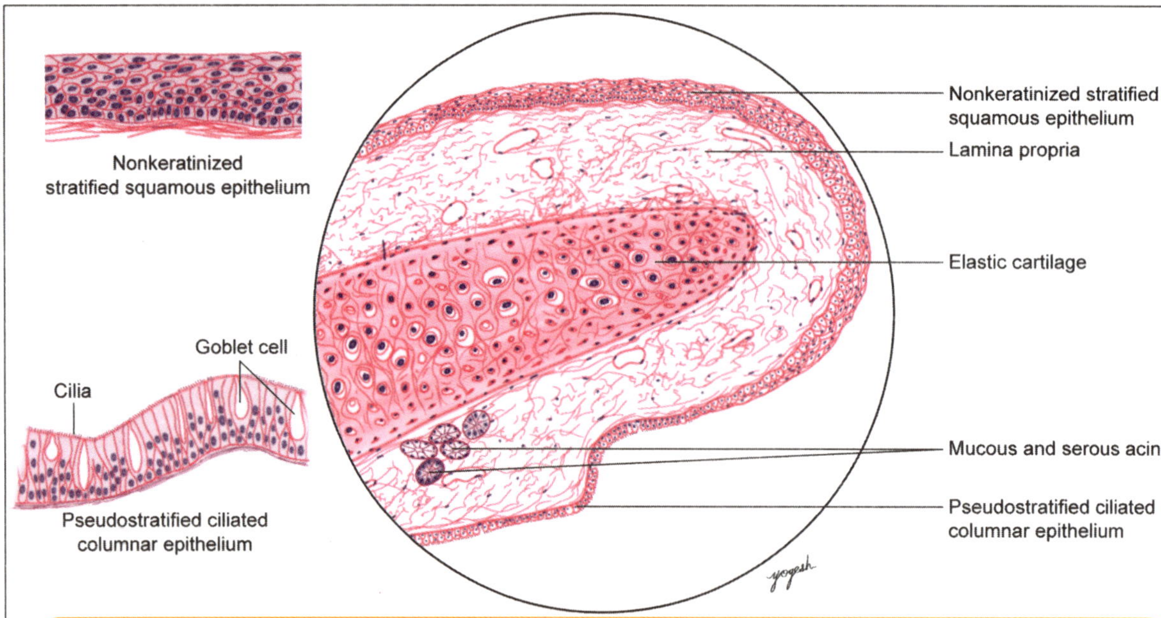


Epiglottis has a core of elastic cartilage covered by mucous membrane.
It is lined by

1. Ciliated pseudostratified columnar epithelium on one side and
2. Nonkeratinized stratified squamous epithelium on another.

Connective tissue is vascular and shows mucous and serous glands.

*Space for Notes*

## Plate 45: **Trachea**

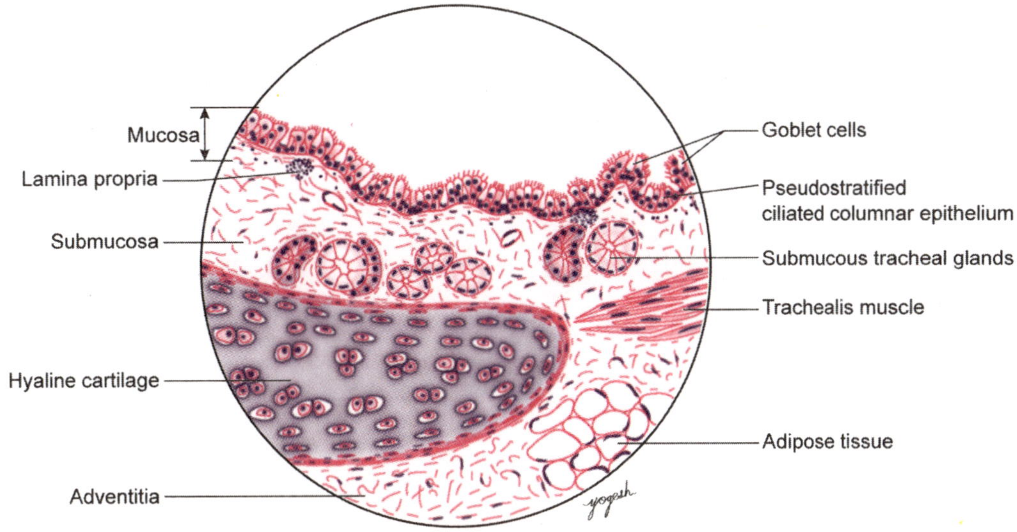


Mucosa has pseudostratified ciliated columnar epithelium with goblet cells.
Epithelium rest on thick basement membrane and lamina propria.
It has a layer of C-shaped hyaline cartilages and trachealis (smooth) muscle.
Externally covered by fibroelastic tissue of adventitia.

## Plate 46: **Lung**

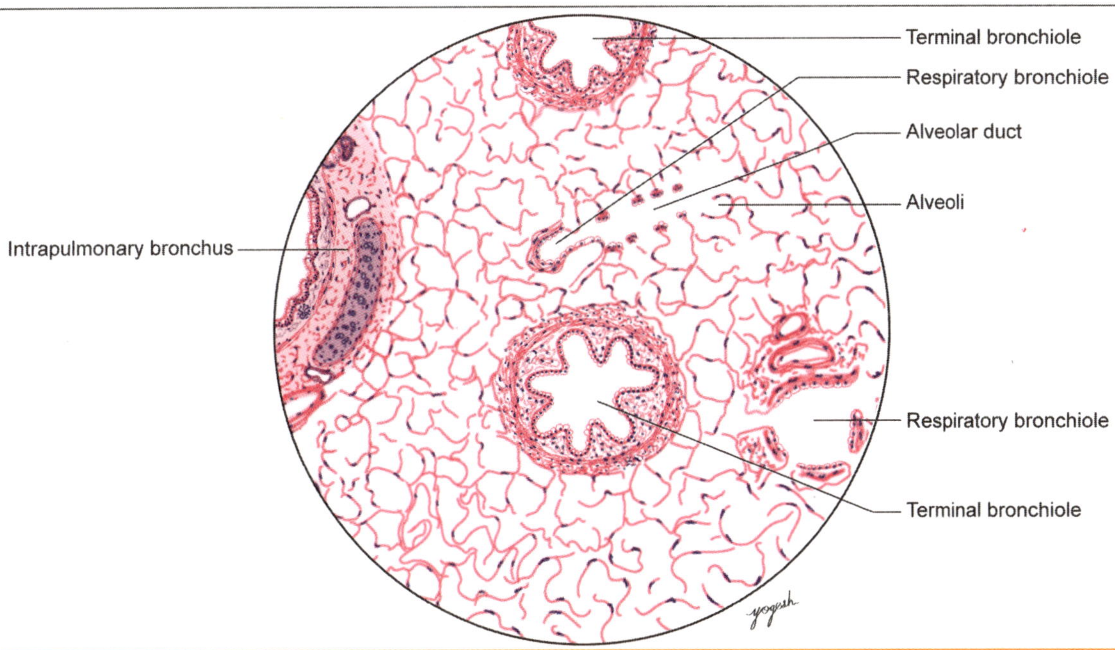


Intrapulmonary bronchi are lined by pseudostratified ciliated columnar epithelium with goblet cells. They have complete circumferential smooth muscle layer and discontinuous cartilaginous plates.
Bronchioles show transition from ciliated pseudostratified columnar epithelium to ciliated columnar and finally simple cuboidal epithelium. Bronchioles do not have cartilage plates.
Respiratory bronchiole has simple cuboidal epithelium and smooth muscles layer.
Alveoli are polyhedral sacs lined by simple squamous epithelium.

*Space for Notes* ____________________

## Plate 47: **Lip**

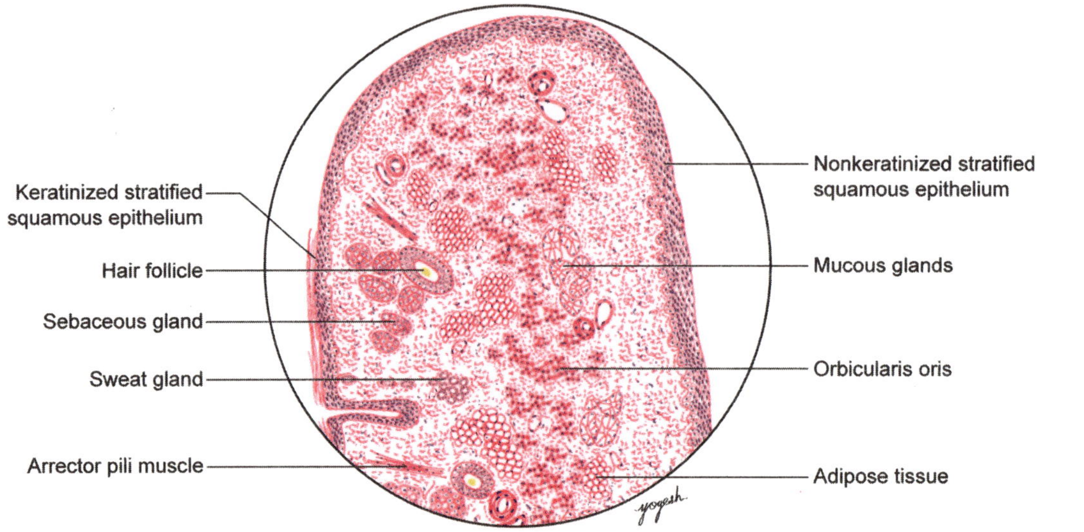


Lip is a mucomuscular fold having core made of skeletal muscles.
It is externally lined by skin and internally by mucous membrane.
Skin covering the lip is lined by stratified squamous epithelium (epidermis), hair follicles, sweat glands, and sebaceous glands.
Mucous membrane of lip is lined by nonkeratinized stratified squamous epithelium.

## Plate 48: **Tooth**

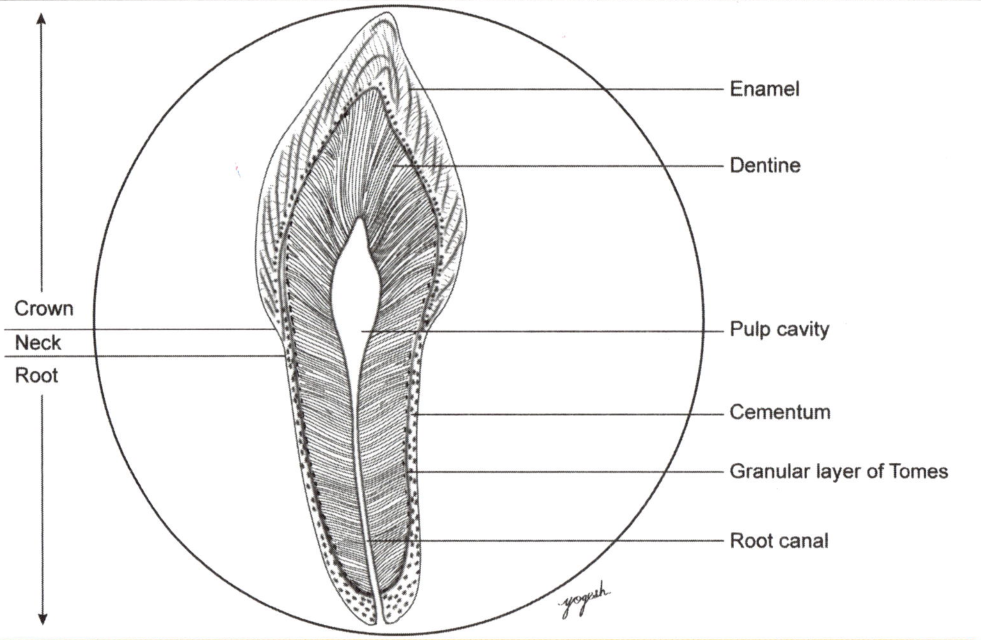


Tooth has three parts: Crown (lies superficial to gum), root (covered by gum and bony alveolar process), and neck (junction of crown and root).
Tooth has four specialized zones/coats:
1. Enamel—covers outer surface of crown of tooth
2. Dentine—lies deep to the enamel in crown and cementum in root
3. Cementum—bone-like calcified tissue in root of tooth
4. Root canal (pulp)—cavity enclosed by dentine

*Space for Notes*

## Plate 49: **Tongue: Anterior Two-thirds**

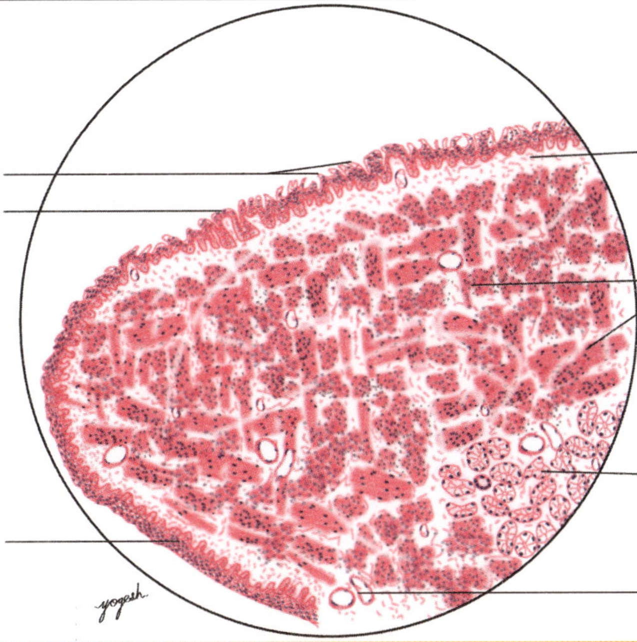


Anterior two-thirds of tongue consists of mucous membrane that covers core of skeletal muscle fibers
Mucous membrane is lined by nonkeratinized stratified squamous epithelium and lamina propria.
Mucosa shows filiform papillae (small, conical projections with keratinized tips) and fungiform papillae (mushroom-shaped projections).
Skeletal muscle fibers in tongue are arranged longitudinally, transversely, and vertically.
Mucous lingual salivary glands are also present.

*Note*: Circumvallate and foliate papillae may be seen. Circumvallate and fungiform papillae show the taste buds.

## Plate 50: **Types of Papillae**

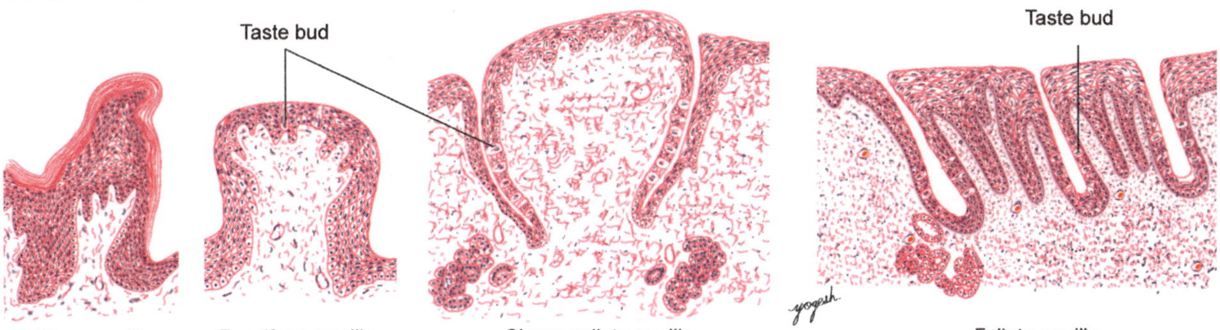


Filiform papilla | Fungiform papilla | Circumvallate papilla | Foliate papilla

*Space for Notes* ____________

Histology Diagrams

## Plate 51: **Tongue: Posterior One-third**

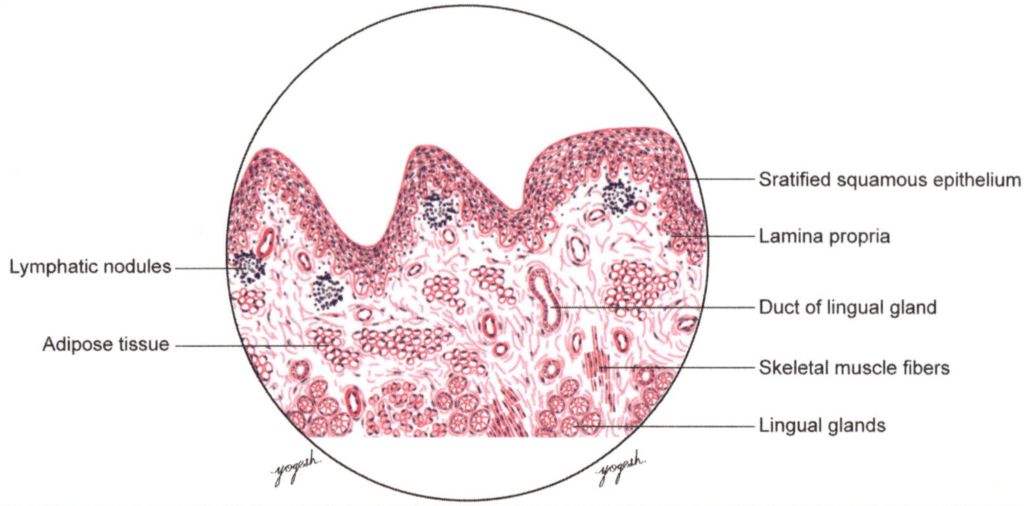


Posterior one-third of tongue consists of mucous membrane (nonkeratinized stratified squamous epithelium and lamina propria) that covers the following structures:
1. Numerous mucous lingual salivary glands and their ducts
2. Lymphatic follicles
3. Core of skeletal muscle fibers (arranged longitudinally, transversely, and vertically).

*Note*: Lingual tonsils are not shown in this figure to avoid the confusion with the histology of palatine tonsil.

## Plate 52: **Esophagus (Lower Part)**

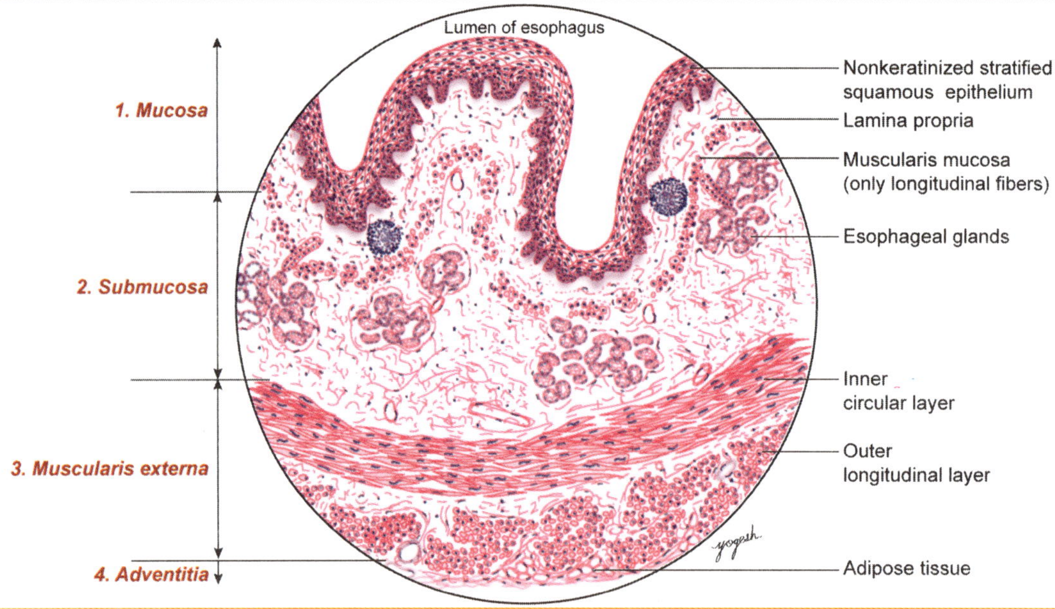


Esophagus has 4 layers: Mucosa, submucosa, muscularis externa, and serosa.
Mucosae has nonkeratinized stratified squamous epithelium, lamina propria, and muscularis mucosa (thick, longitudinal smooth muscles).
Submucosa has compound tubuloalveolar mucous glands.
Muscularis externa has inner circular and outer longitudinal smooth muscle fibers.

*Note*: In upper one-third, wall of esophagus shows skeletal muscles in muscularis externa; in middle third, both skeletal and smooth muscles; whereas in lower-third only smooth muscles are present.

*Space for Notes* __________

## Plate 53: **Gastro-esophageal Junction**

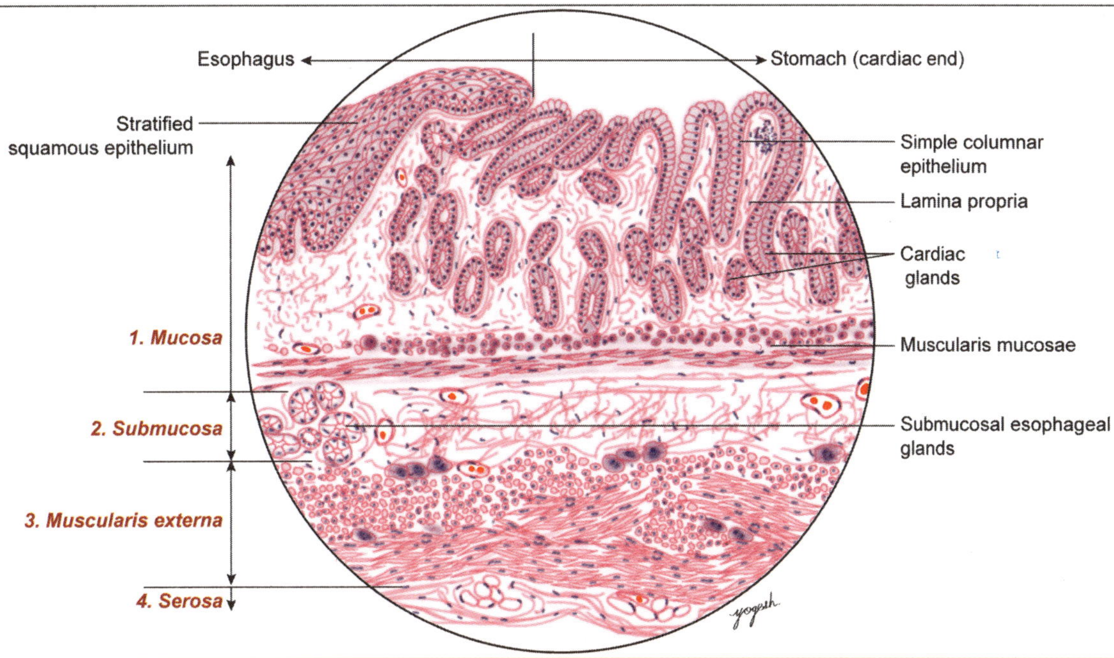


Gastroesophageal junction shows four layers: Mucosa, submucosa, muscularis externa, and serosa/adventitia.
Esophagus shows nonkeratinized stratified squamous epithelium submucosal compound tubuloalveolar glands.
Cardiac part of stomach is lined by surface mucous cells (simple columnar cells) and has cardiac glands with mucus-secreting cells.
The junction is marked by transition zone of epithelium.

## Plate 54: **Stomach: Fundus and Body**

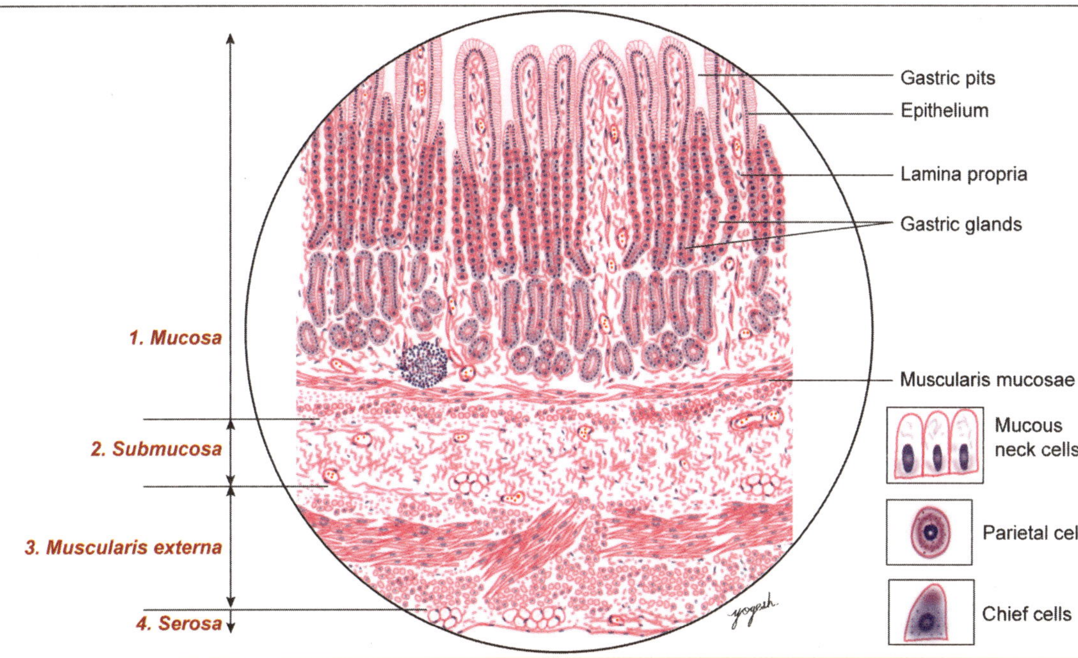


Stomach shows four layers: Mucosa, submucosa, muscularis externa, and serosa.
Mucosa is lined by surface mucous cells (simple columnar cells).
Mucosa shows short gastric pits and long branched tubular glands gastric glands with pink oxyntic cells (HCl, intrinsic factor), neck mucous cells (mucus), and blue-colored deeper chief cells (pepsinogen).
Muscularis externa has randomly oriented smooth muscle cells (inner oblique, middle circular, and outer longitudinal layers).

*Space for Notes* ____________________

## Plate 55: **Stomach: Pylorus**

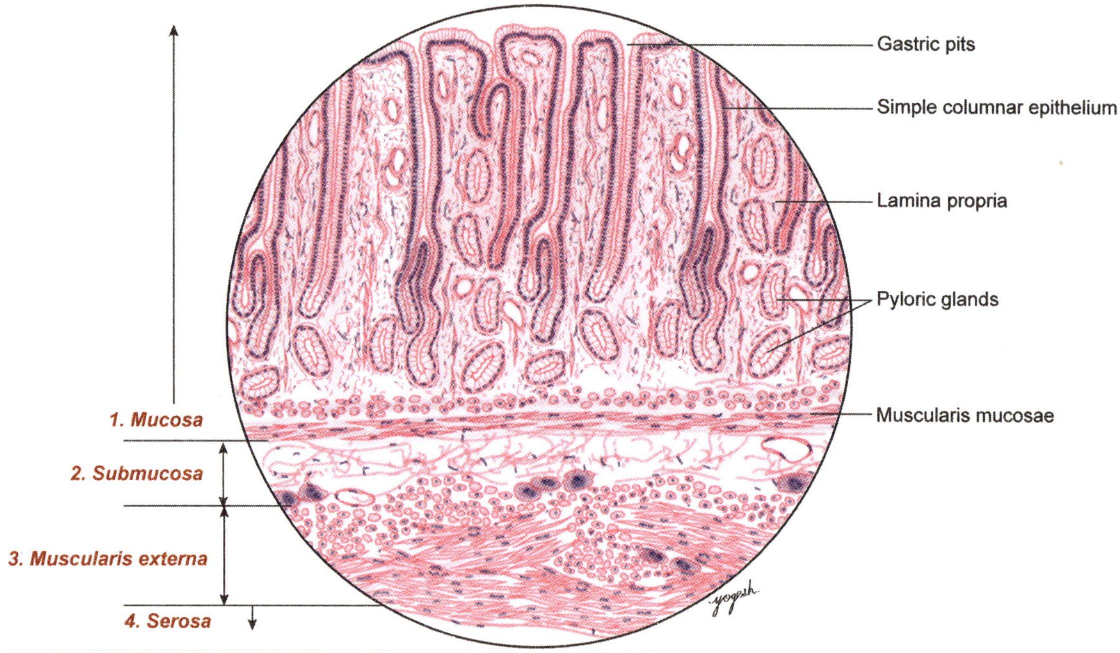


Stomach shows four layers: Mucosa, submucosa, muscularis externa, and serosa.
Mucosa is lined by surface mucous cells (simple columnar cells).
Mucosa shows long gastric pits and short branched tubular glands gastric glands (lined by mucus-secreting cells).
Muscularis externa has thick circular smooth muscle fibers form pyloric sphincter.

## Plate 56: **Duodenum**

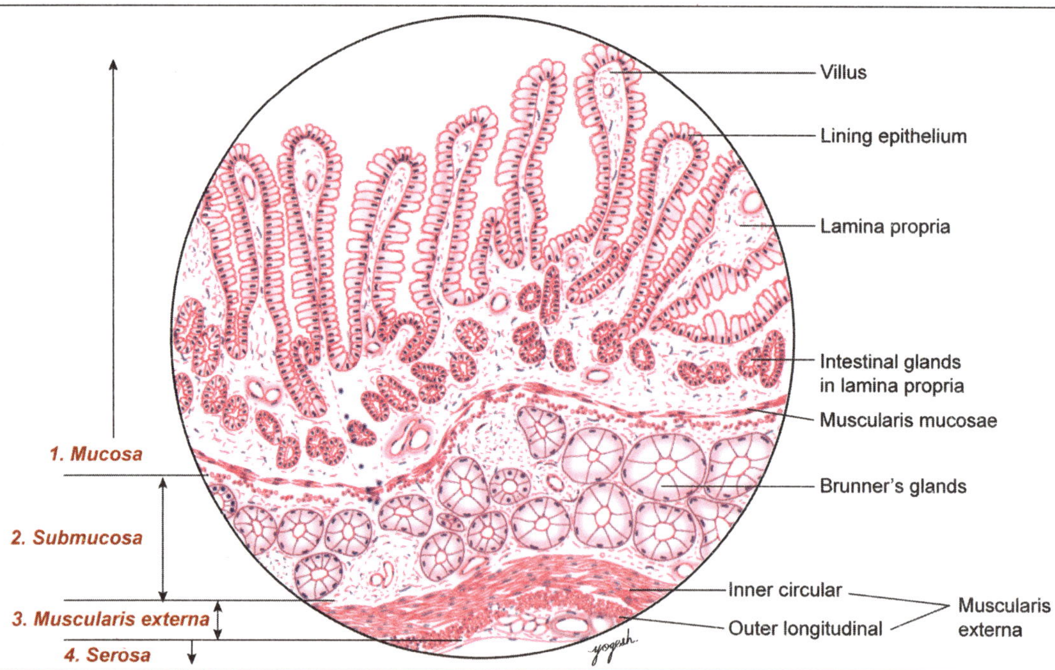


Duodenum has four layers: Mucosa, submucosa, muscularis externa, and serosa/adventitia.
Finger-like villi lined by simple columnar epithelium with striated border because of microvilli and few goblet cells.
Crypts of Lieberkühn/intestinal glands are present in lamina propria above muscularis mucosa.
***Brunner's glands*** are highly branched, tubuloalveolar mixed glands that are located in submucosa.
Muscularis externa has inner circular and outer longitudinal smooth muscle layers.

*Space for Notes*

## Plate 57: **Jejunum**

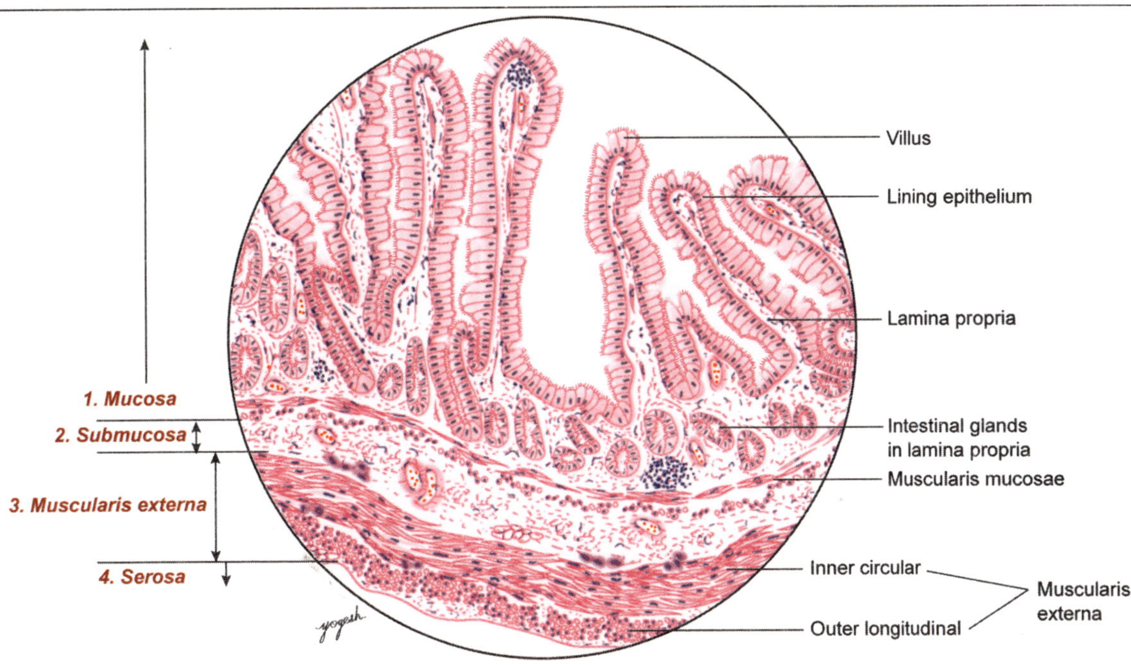


Jejunum has four layers: Mucosa, submucosa, muscularis externa, and serosa.
It shows tongue-shaped villi (lined with simple columnar epithelium and striated border), and intestinal glands.
Brunner's glands and Peyer's patches are ***absent***.
Muscularis externa has inner circular and outer longitudinal smooth muscle layers.

## Plate 58: **Ileum**

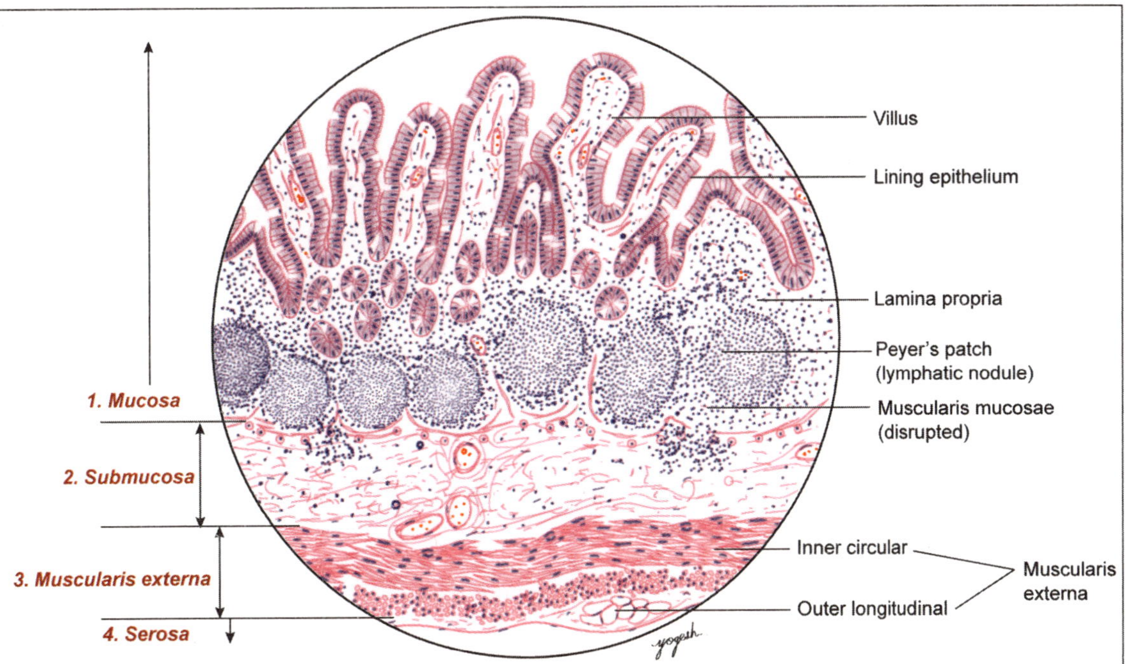


Ileum has four layers: Mucosa, submucosa, muscularis externa, and serosa/adventitia.
It has few, short, finger-like villi (mucosal projections with a core of lamina propria) lined with simple columnar epithelium with striated border (microvilli) and goblet cells.
Lamina propria contains intestinal glands and Peyer's patches.
Muscularis mucosa is thin and even absent at the site of large Peyer's patches.

*Space for Notes*

## Plate 59: **Large Intestine**

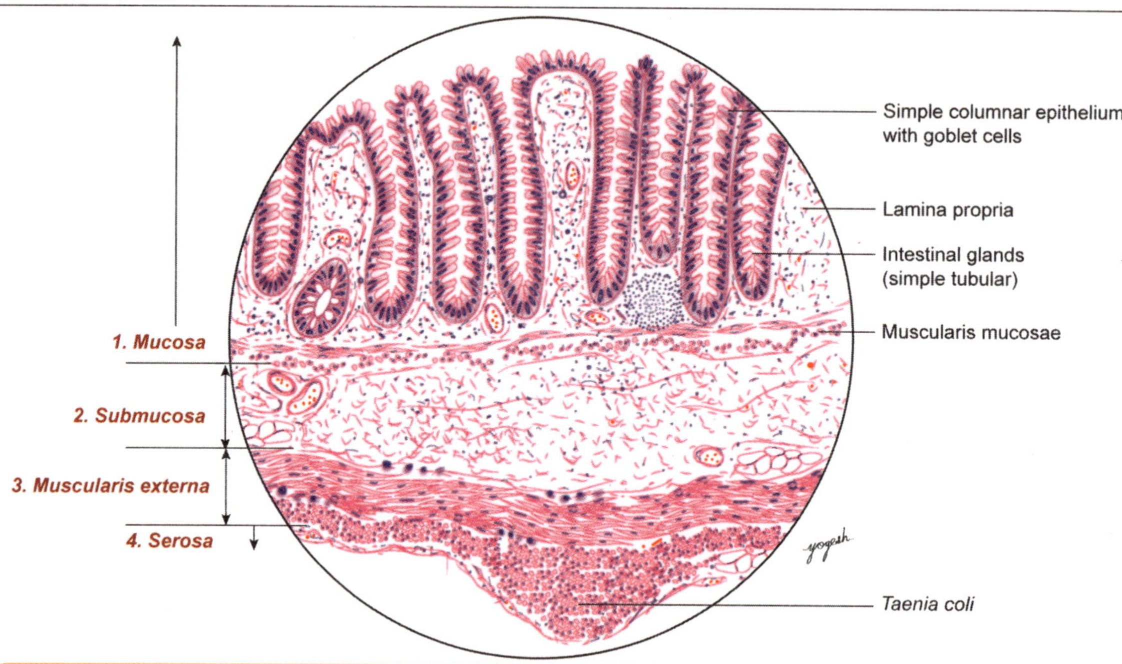


Colon shows four layers: Mucosa, submucosa, muscularis externa, and serosa.
Mucosa is lined by simple columnar epithelium with microvilli and goblet cells.
Lamina propria is filled with intestinal glands that are lined by simple columnar epithelium with goblet cells.
Muscularis externa has inner circular and outer longitudinal fibers. Longitudinal fibers form three bands of *taenia coli*.
Plicae cicrularis, villi, and Paneth cells are absent in large intestine.

## Plate 60: **Appendix**

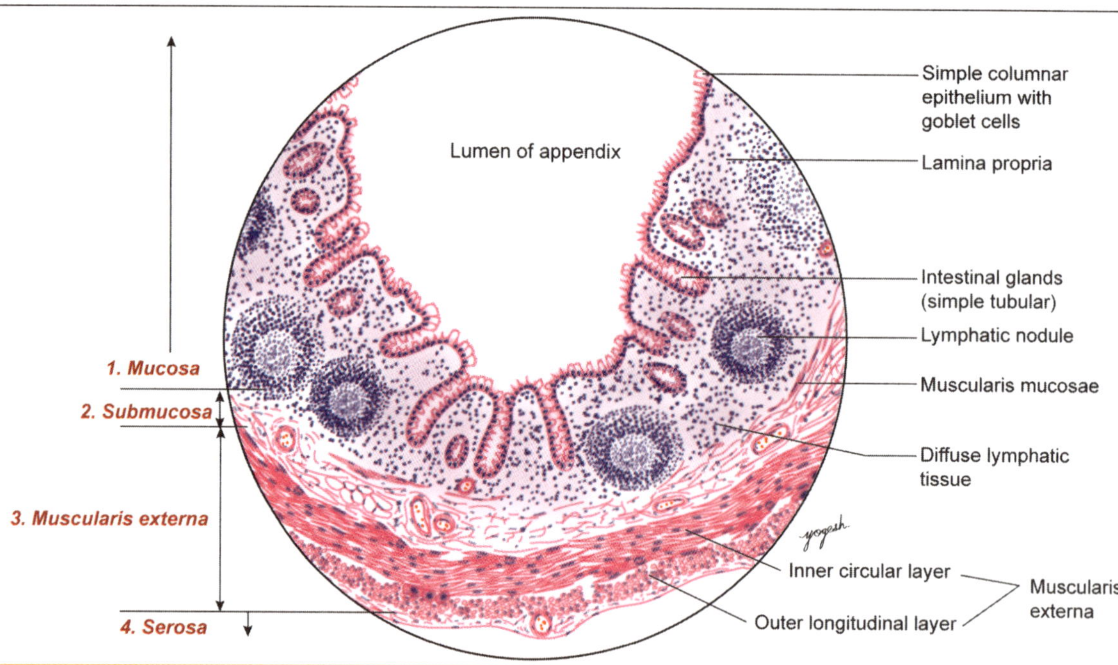


Appendix has four layers: Mucosa, submucosa, muscularis externa, and serosa.
Mucosa is lined by simple columnar epithelium with microvilli and numerous goblet cells.
Lamina propria contains simple tubular intestinal glands lined by simple columnar epithelium with goblet cells.
Lamina propria is occupied by lymphatic follicles that may even may cross muscularis mucosa and extend into submucosa.

*Space for Notes* ______________________________

## Plate 61: **Liver**

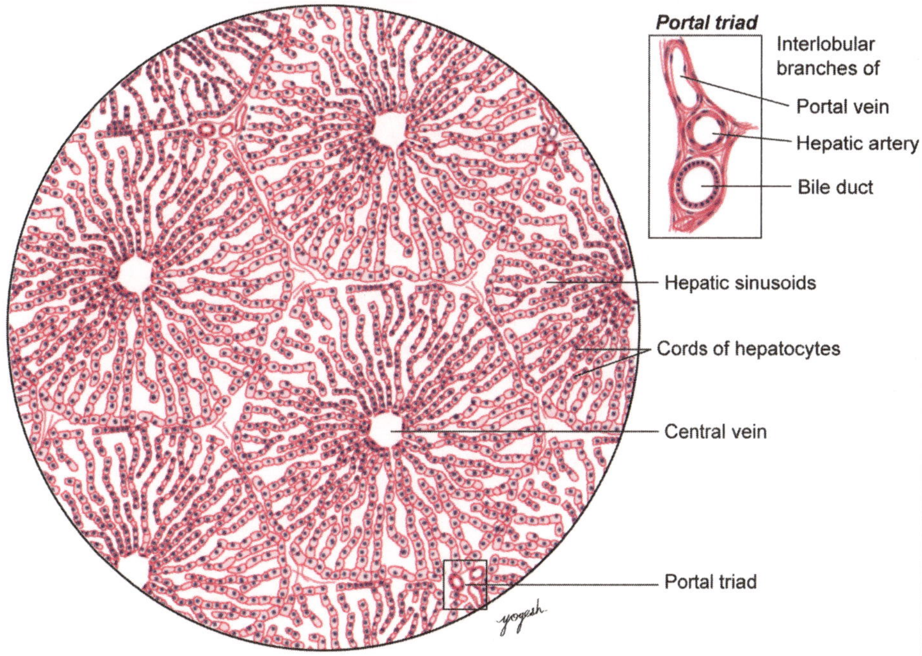


Liver shows hexagonal classical hepatic lobules. Central vein lies in the form of space at the center of lobule.
Cords of hepatocytes—arranged radially, radiating away from central vein. Liver sinusoids separate cords of hepatocytes.
Portal triad consists of

1. Branch of portal vein (simple squamous epithelium)
2. Branch of hepatic artery (simple squamous epithelium), and
3. Interlobular bile duct (simple cuboidal to columnar epithelium).

## Plate 62: **Gallbladder**

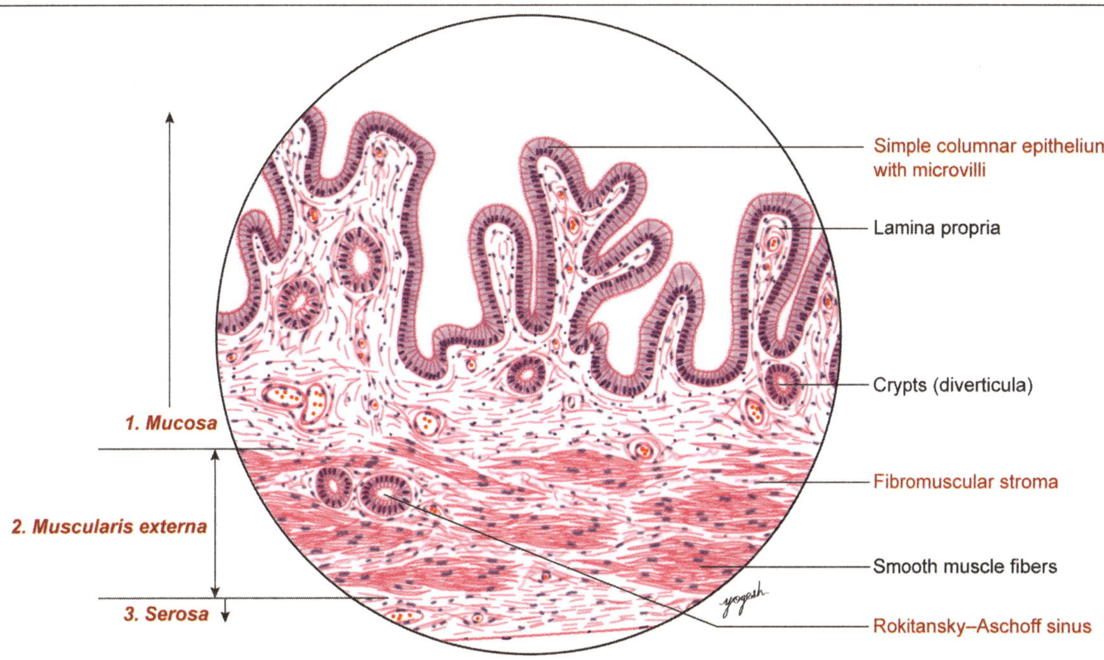


Gallbladder shows three layers:

1. Mucosa is lined by tall columnar cells with striated border (microvilli) and lamina propria
2. Fibromuscular coat consists of bundle of smooth muscle fibers with interspaced collagen and elastic fibers.
3. Serosa/adventitia

Note: Gallbladder does not have villi, goblet cells, submucosa, and properly organized muscularis externa.

*Space for Notes* __________

## Plate 63: **Pancreas**

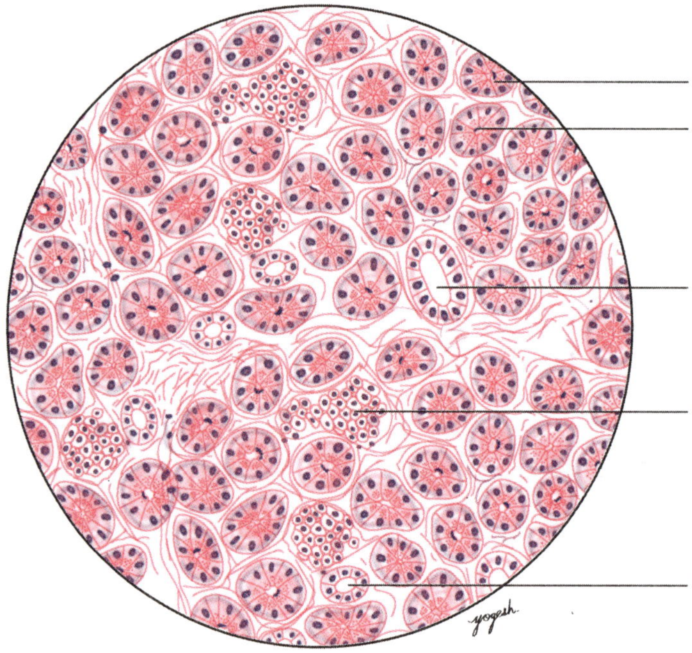


Pancreas shows exocrine as well as endocrine components.
Exocrine pancreas (serous compound tubuloalveolar part) consists of serous acini that are lined by tall columnar cells and centroacinar cells (simple squamous cells).
Interlobular ducts are lined by simple cuboidal to low columnar epithelium.
Endocrine pancreas (islets of Langerhans) are lightly stained clusters of polygonal cells.

## Plate 64: **Kidney**

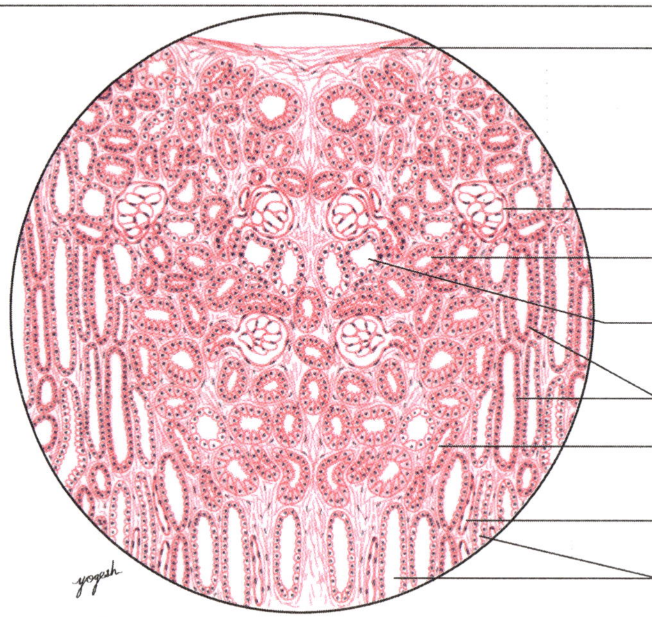


Kidney has outer cortex and inner medulla and is covered by a connective tissue capsule.
Kidney shows presence of renal corpuscles and renal tubules.
Renal corpuscle consists of glomeruli, Bowman's capsule, Bowman's space.

Renal tubules:
- Proximal convoluted tubules (PCT) (simple cuboidal epithelium with prominent brush border)
- Proximal straight tubule (simple cuboidal epithelium with microvilli)
- Loop of Henle: thin segment (simple squamous epithelium), thick segment (cuboidal epithelium)
- Distal convoluted tubules (DCT) (simple cuboidal epithelium)
- Collecting tubules and ducts (simple cuboidal to columnar epithelium).

*Space for Notes*

## Plate 65: **Ureter**

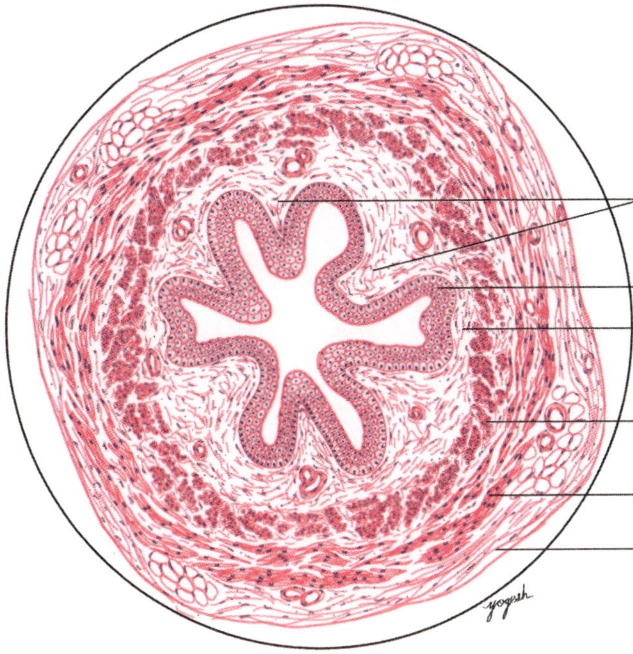


Ureter is mucomuscular tube with star-shaped lumen.
It has three layers:

- Inner mucous membrane lined by transitional epithelium and lamina propria.
- Middle smooth muscle layer
- Outer adventitia (connective tissue coat)

## Plate 66: **Urinary Bladder**

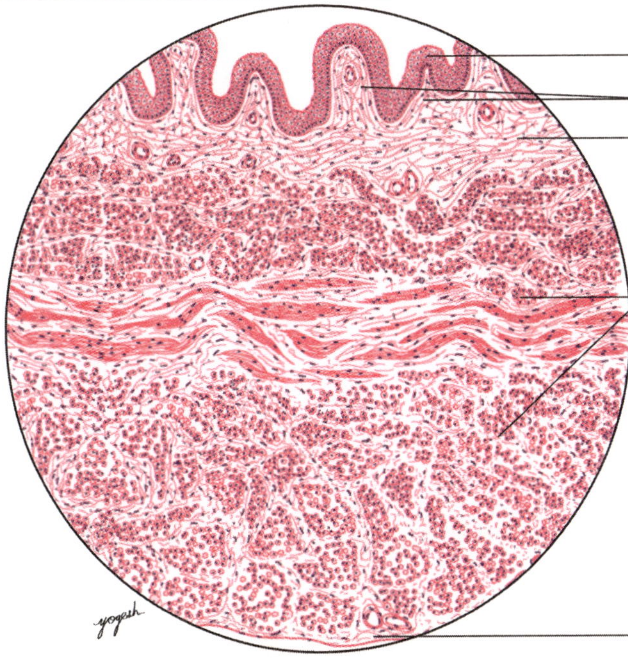


It has three layers: Inner mucous layer, middle thick smooth muscle coat, and outer serous layer.
Interior of urinary bladder is lined by 3–6-cell-layered thick transitional epithelium covered by thick eosinophilic plaques.
Transitional epithelium rests on thick coat of lamina propria.
It has thick muscle coat with inner and outer layers arranged longitudinally, and middle run obliquely.

*Space for Notes* ____________________

## Plate 67: **Testis**

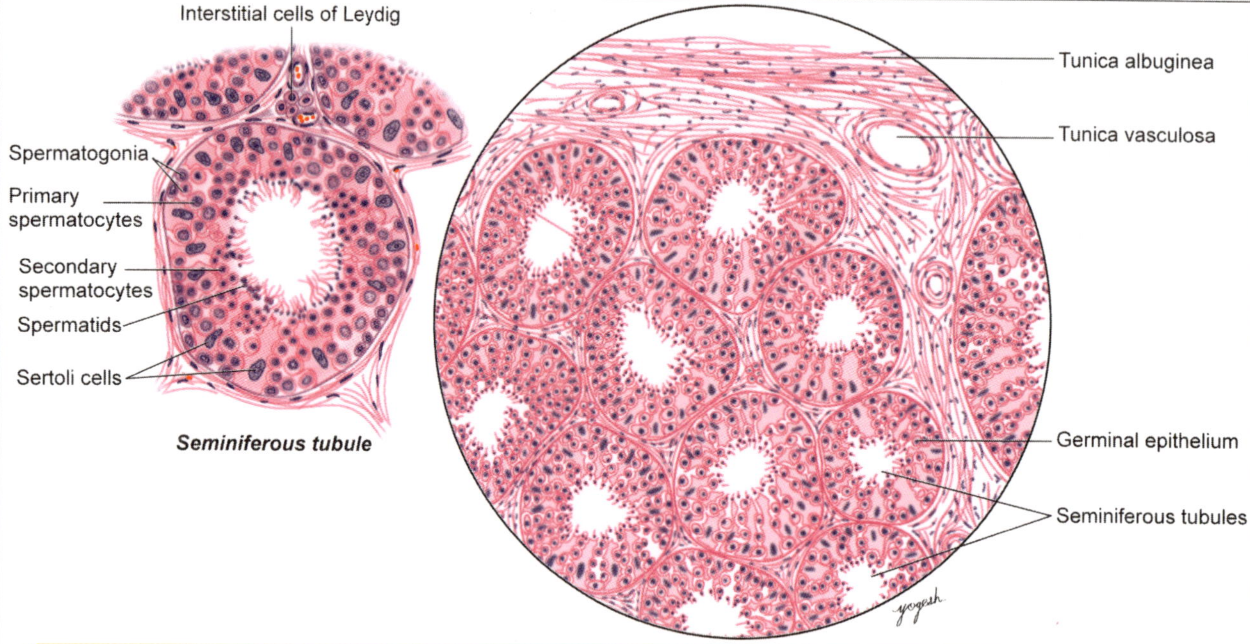


Testis is covered by fibrous tunica albuginea and vascular tunica vasculosa.
Testis has seminiferous tubules that are surrounded by lamina propria.
Seminiferous tubules are lined by seminiferous epithelium with two types of cells: Spermatogenic cells (spermatogonia, spermatids, and sperms) and tall, columnar Sertoli cells.
Leydig (interstitial) cells are polyhedral eosinophilic cells that lie in clusters surrounding the seminiferous tubules.

## Plate 68: **Epididymis**

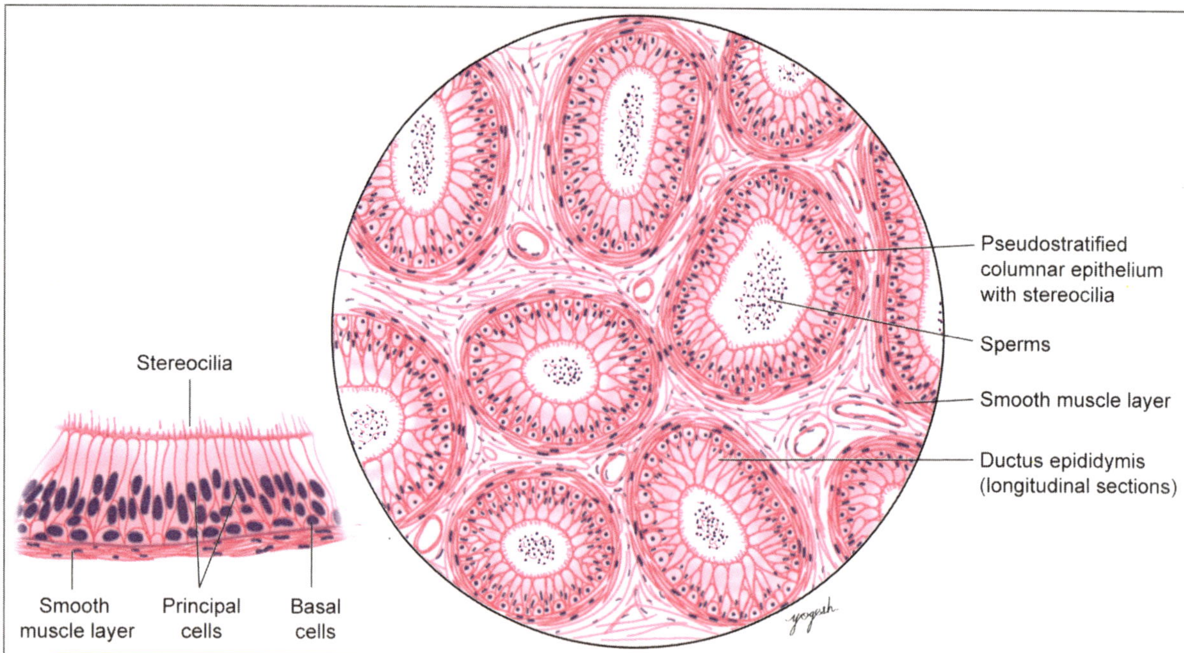


Epididymis has a single, highly coiled duct of epididymis lined by pseudostratified columnar epithelium. It has tall principal cells with numerous stereocilia and short basal cells.
Muscle coat consists of thin layers of circular smooth muscle cells.

*Space for Notes* ____________________

## Plate 69: **Ductus Deferens/Vas Deferens**

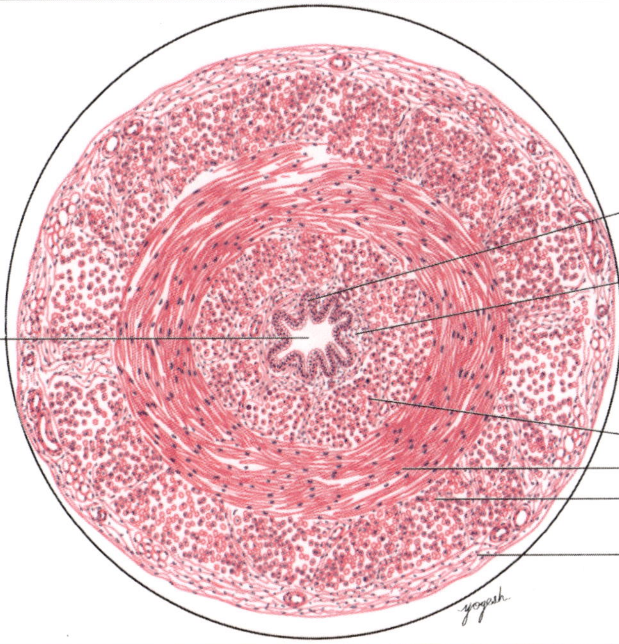


Vas deferens is a thick-walled muscular tube (star-shaped lumen) having three layers:

- Mucosa—Lined by pseudostratified columnar epithelium with nonmotile cilia.
- Smooth muscle coat arranged as inner and outer longitudinal and middle thick circular layers
- Adventitia consists of loose areolar tissue

***Function***

Ejaculation of sperms

## Plate 70: **Seminal Vesicle**

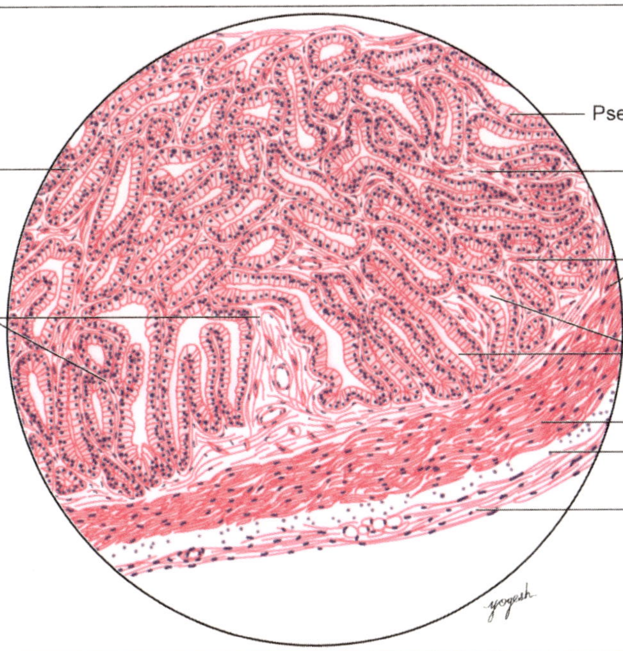


Seminal vesicle has three layers:

- Mucosa: Lined by pseudostratified columnar epithelium resting on lamina propria.
- Mucosa is highly folded and occupies most of the lumen.
- Smooth muscle coat: Arranged as inner circular and outer longitudinal layers.
- Adventitia: Loose connective tissue.

***Function***

Secretion of fructose-rich, alkaline seminal fluid

*Space for Notes*

## Plate 71: **Prostate**

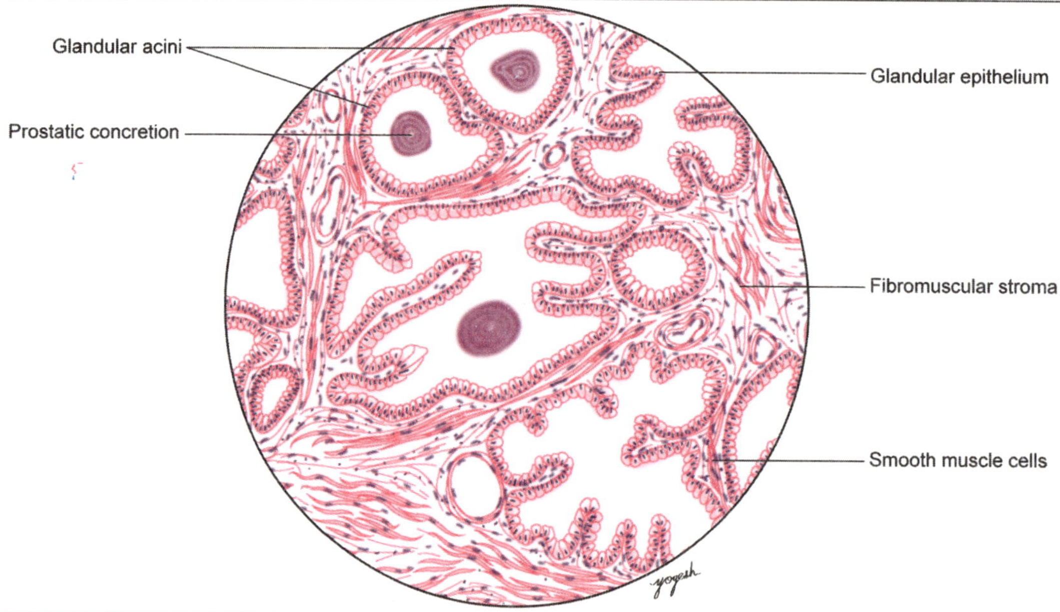


Prostate consists of 30–50 tubuloalveolar glands.
- Mucosa: lined by Simple columnar to pseudostratified columnar epithelium and thrown into folds.
- Fibromuscular stroma contains smooth muscles, collagen fibers, and elastic fibers.
- ***Corpora amylasea***: Concentric lamellated eosinophilic structures in prostatic alveoli in old age.

***Function***

Secretion of prostatic fluid (contains fibrinolysin and prostate-specific antigen)

## Plate 72: **Penis**

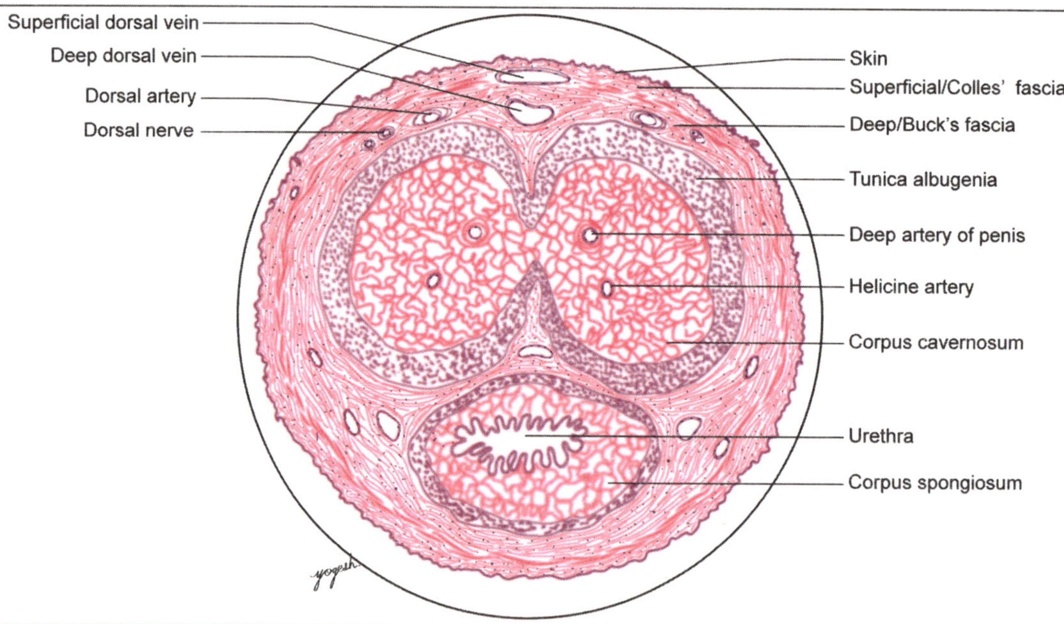


Penis consists of three masses of erectile tissues:
- Two dorsal corpora cavernosa: contains numerous vascular spaces and covered by thin smooth muscle layer.
- A single ventral corpus spongiosum: Sponge-like tissue that surrounds the penile urethra.

Tunica albuginea is a thick connective tissue sheath that is covered by a thin layer of connective tissue (devoid of fat) and skin (devoid of hairs).

Penile urethra is lined by pseudostratified columnar epithelium (except at terminal part—by stratified squamous epithelium).

*Space for Notes* ___

## Plate 73: **Ovary**

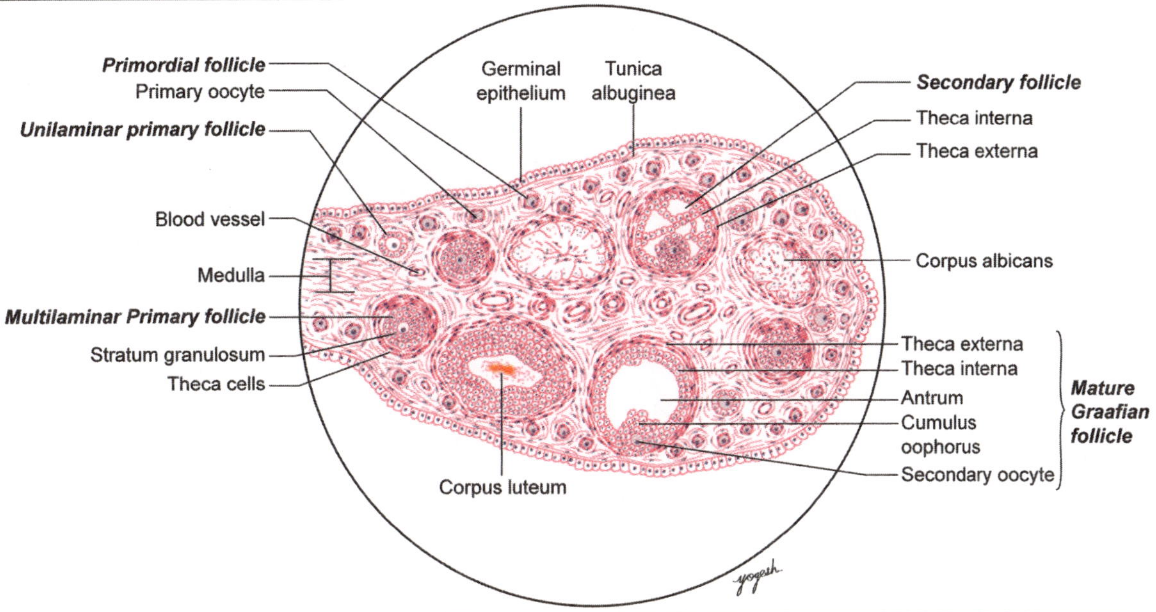


Ovary has 1. Inner medulla that consists of connective tissue, blood vessels, and nerves; 2. Outer cortex that shows follicles of various sizes; 3. Tunica albuginea (connective tissue layer); and 4. Outermost cuboidal germinal epithelium.
Primordial follicle: Primary oocyte covered by a flattened layer of follicular cells.
Primary follicle: Primary oocyte covered by zona pellucida and single or multi-layered cell thick cuboidal follicular cells.
Secondary follicle: Primary oocyte is covered by zona pellucida, granulosa cells with follicular antrum, theca interna (vascular), and theca externa (fibrous) layers. Graafian follicle: It shows secondary oocyte. Corpus luteum: Consists of luteal cells.
Corpus albicans: Fibrous tissue.

## Plate 74: **Uterus: Proliferative Phase**

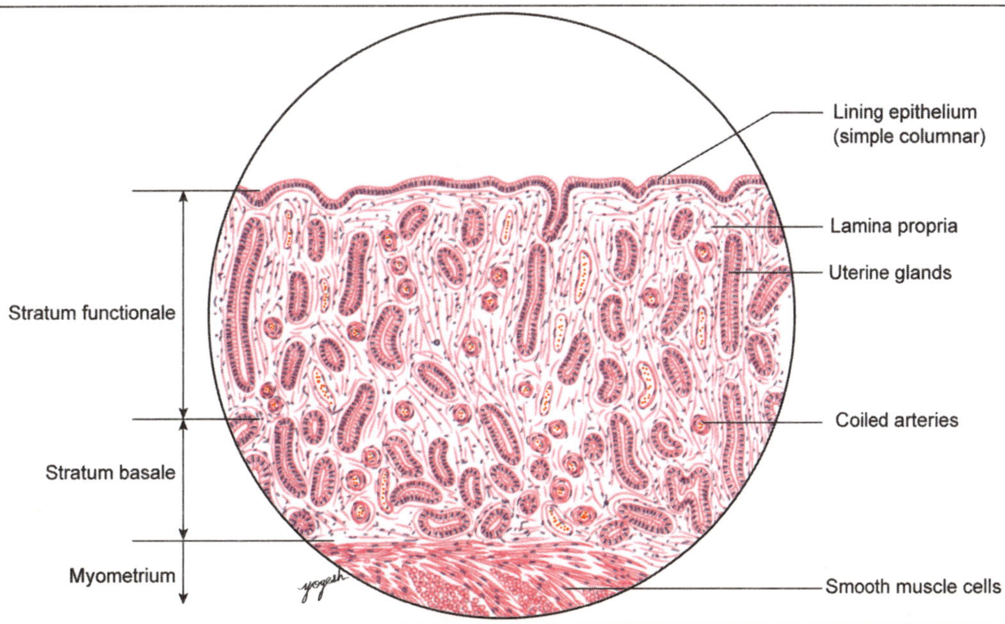


Uterus has three layers:

1. Inner endometrium consists of simple columnar epithelial lining, simple tubular glands and spiral arteries.
2. Middle thick myometrium consists of smooth muscle cells.
3. Perimetrium consists of connective tissue layer covered by mesothelium.

In ***proliferative phase***: Glands are long with narrow lumen; thick stroma with less coiled spiral arteries.

*Space for Notes* ___

## Plate 75: **Uterus: Secretory Phase**

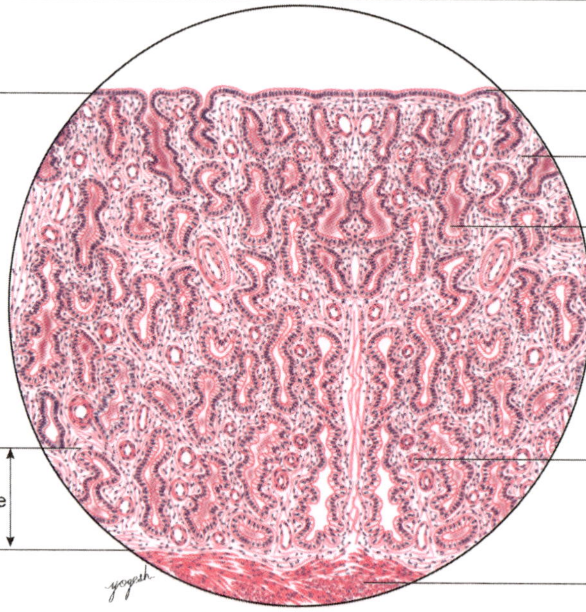


Uterus three layers:

1. Inner endometrium consists of simple columnar epithelial lining, simple tubular glands and spiral arteries.
2. Middle thick myometrium consists of smooth muscle cells.
3. Outer perimetrium: Connective tissue layer.

In secretory phase: Glands are highly coiled with wide lumen and secretions, stroma with coiled spiral arteries.

## Plate 76: **Cervix of Uterus**

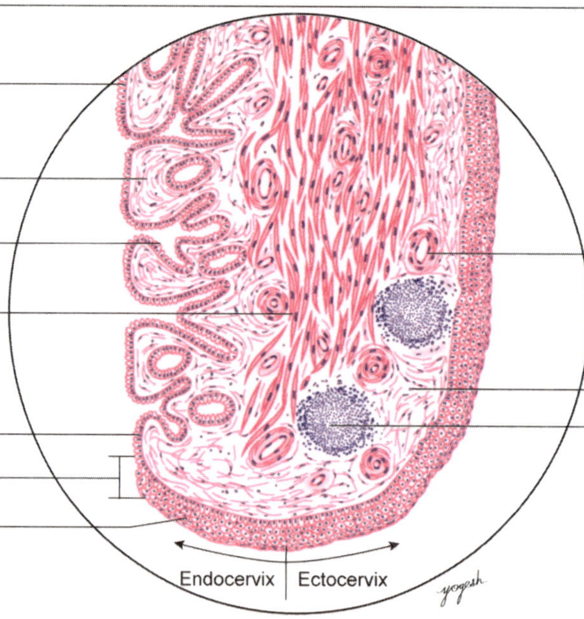


Cervix of uterus shows

Endocervix—Lined by tall columnar mucus secreting epithelium that rests on lamina propria (loose areolar tissue).

Cervical glands are small, branched tubular glands in lamina propria.

Muscle coat of smooth muscle fibers

Ectocervix/Portio vaginalis—Portion of cervix that projects into the vagina and lined by stratified squamous epithelium.

*Space for Notes* ________________

## Plate 77: **Fallopian Tube**

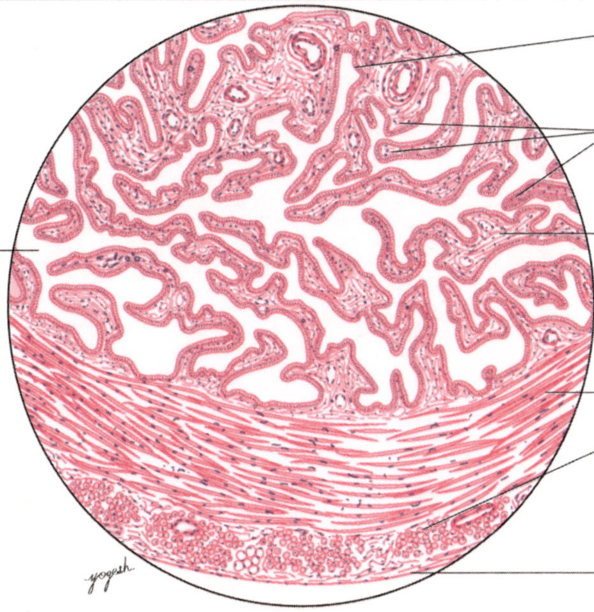


Fallopian tube shows three layers from inside outwards:
- Mucosa consists of thin projecting longitudinal folds that fill the lumen. These folds are lined by ciliated simple columnar epithelium (with peg cells and intercalary cells)
- Muscle layer consists of inner thick circular and outer thin longitudinal smooth muscle cell layers.
- Serosa—covered by a simple squamous epithelium.

## Plate 78: **Mammary Gland: Inactive Stage**

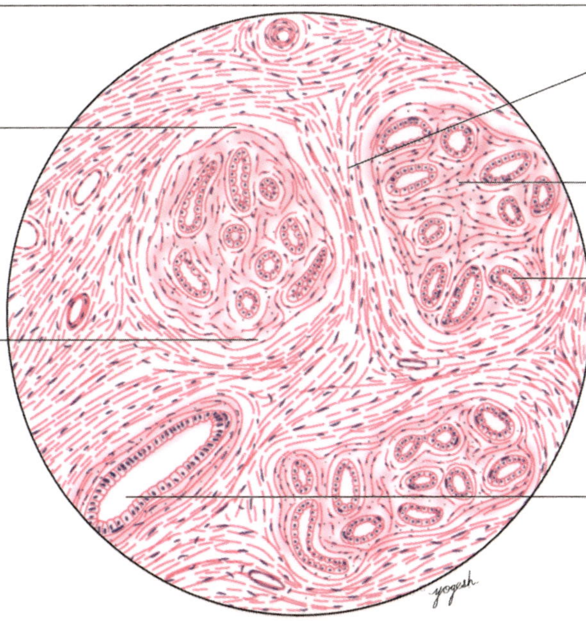


Mammary gland is composed of ducts, parenchyma, and stroma.
Parenchyma: Each gland shows 15–20 lobes of compound tubuloalveolar gland.
Nonlactating inactive glands: Shows spherical masses or cords of alveolar cells.
Ducts: Lactiferous duct: Lined by columnar epithelium; Interlobular ducts: Lined by cuboidal to low columnar epithelium.
Intralobular ducts: Lined by cuboidal epithelium; Alveolar ducts: Lined by low cuboidal epithelium.
Stroma: More connective tissue.

*Space for Notes* ________________

## Plate 79: **Mammary Gland: In lactation**

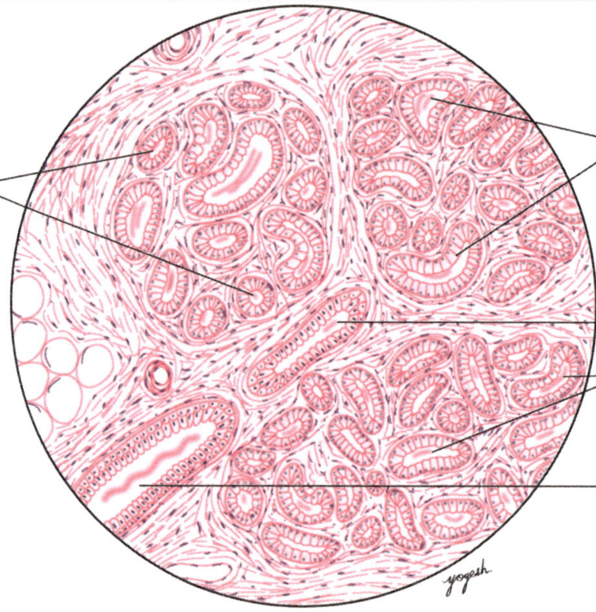


Mammary gland is composed of ducts, parenchyma, and stroma.
Parenchyma: Each gland shows 15–20 lobes of compound tubuloalveolar gland.
Lactating active glands: Shows numerous branched ducts with clusters of alveoli that are lined by simple columnar epithelium
Ducts: Lactiferous duct: Lined by columnar epithelium; Interlobular ducts: Lined by cuboidal to low columnar epithelium.
Intralobular ducts: Lined by cuboidal epithelium; Alveolar ducts: Lined by low cuboidal epithelium.
Stroma: Consists of connective tissue.

## Plate 80: **Placenta**

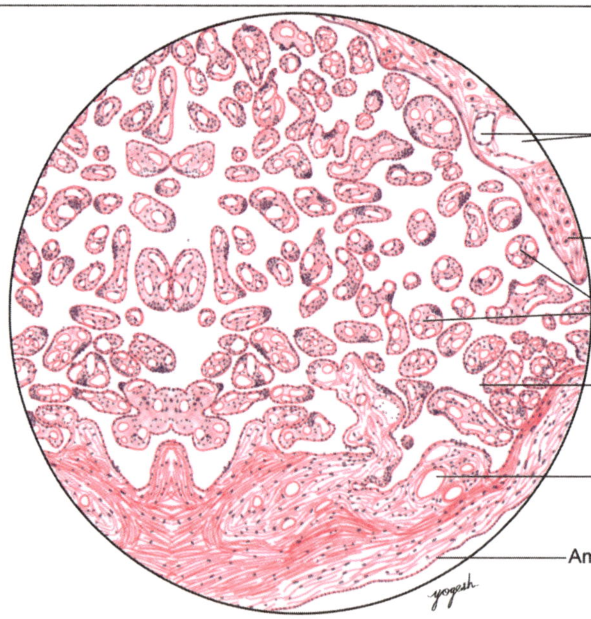


Placenta has chorionic plate that consists of amnion (cuboidal epithelium), connective tissue layer, and fetal blood vessels.
It also has basal plate that shows connective tissue, decidual cells, and placental septa.
Core of placenta consists of chorionic villi and intervillous spaces.
Chorionic villi show outer syncytiotrophoblasts (multinucleated protoplasm), occasional cytotrophoblast, connective tissue, and fetal vessels.
Intervillous spaces are filled with maternal blood.

*Space for Notes* ____

## Plate 81: **Umbilical Cord**

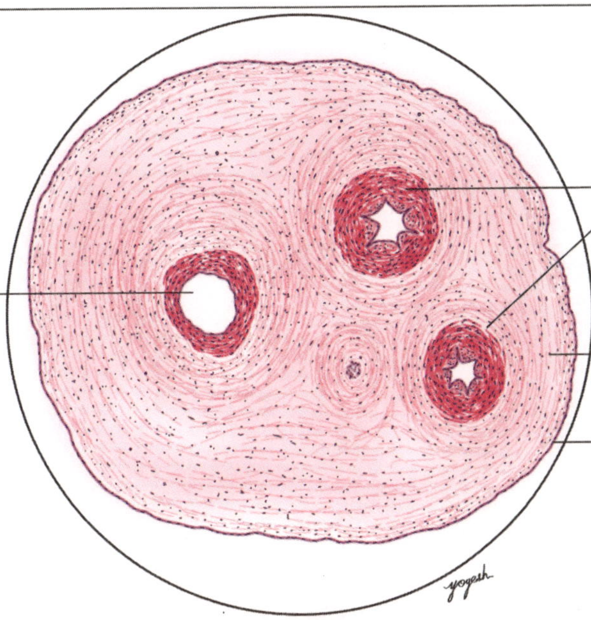


Umbilical cord consists of two umbilical arteries and one umbilical vein embedded in Wharton's jelly.
Umbilical artery has numerous subendothelial cushions whereas umbilical vein do not have subendothelial cushions.
Lumen of umbilical artery is star-shaped, whereas lumen of umbilical vein is wide (oval).
Wharton's jelly is a mucoid connective tissue that has fibroblasts, collagen fibers, and extracellular matrix.

## Plate 82: **Pituitary Gland**

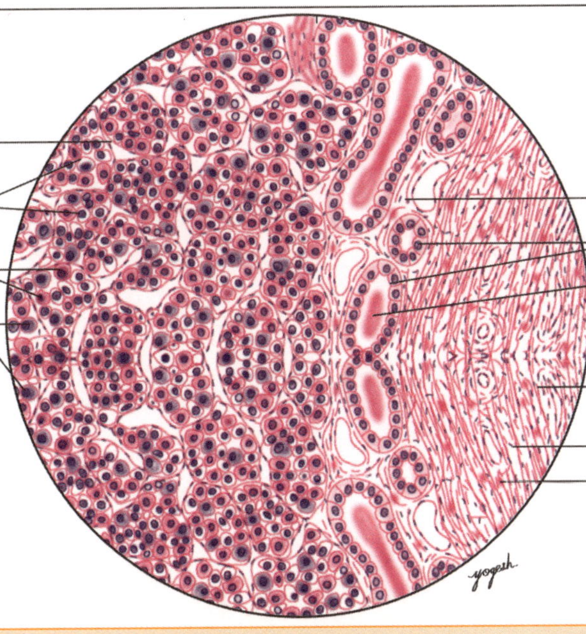


Pituitary gland consists of
Adenohypophysis: It shows clumps or cords of cells separated by fenestrated capillaries. These cells consist of:
- Acidophils: Having pink granules (somatotrophs—secrete growth hormone; lactotropes—secrete prolactin) and
- Basophils: Having dark blue granules (corticotropes—secrete ACTH; gonadotropes—secrete LH and FSH; thyrotropes—secrete TSH)

Pars intermedia consists of a series of colloid-filled cysts/vesicles that secrete MSH.
Neurohypophysis consists of nonmyelinated axons and pituicytes. Neurohypophysis secretes vasopressin/ADH and oxytocin.

*Space for Notes* __________

## Plate 83: **Suprarenal/Adrenal Gland**

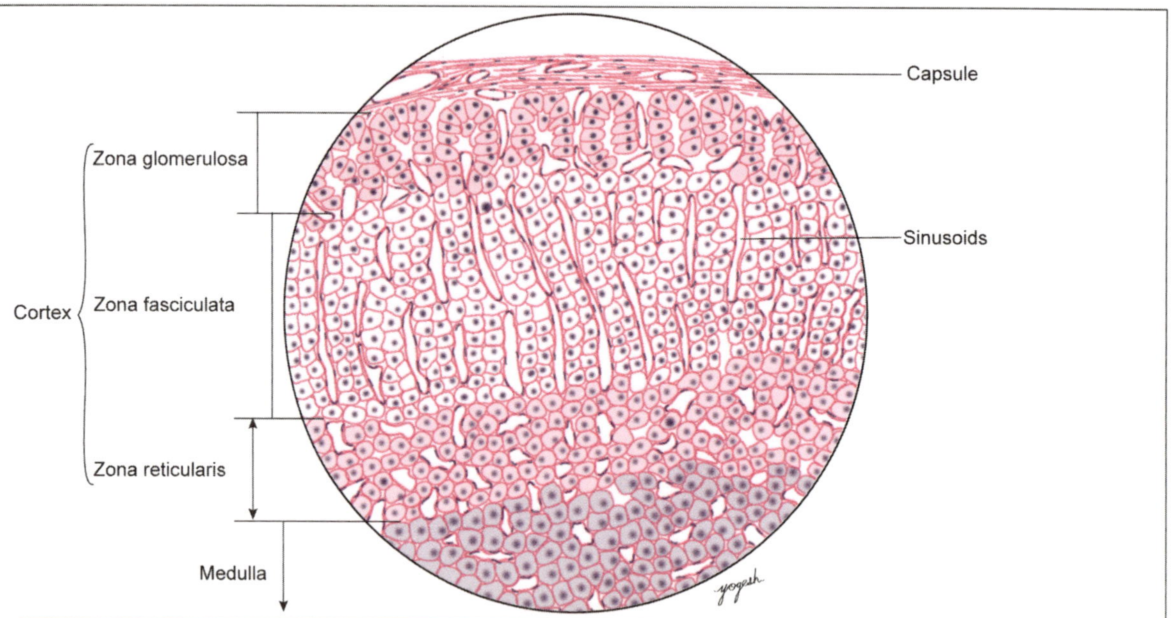


Adrenal gland is surrounded by thick connective tissue capsule, outer cortex, and inner medulla.
Adrenal cortex shows
Outer zona glomerulosa (15%): Ovoid clusters or curved columns of small acidophilic cells.
Middle zona fasciculata (80%): Long straight columns of large polyhedral light-pink cells separated by sinusoidal capillaries.
Inner zona reticularis (5%): Anastomosing cords of small cells separated by fenestrated capillaries.
Adrenal medulla consists of ovoid groups of pale-staining epithelioid cells and blood vessels.
Secretions: Zona glomerulosa—mineralocorticoids; Zona fasciculata—glucocorticoids; Zona reticularis—weak androgens; Adrenal medulla—catecholamines

## Plate 84: **Thyroid Gland**

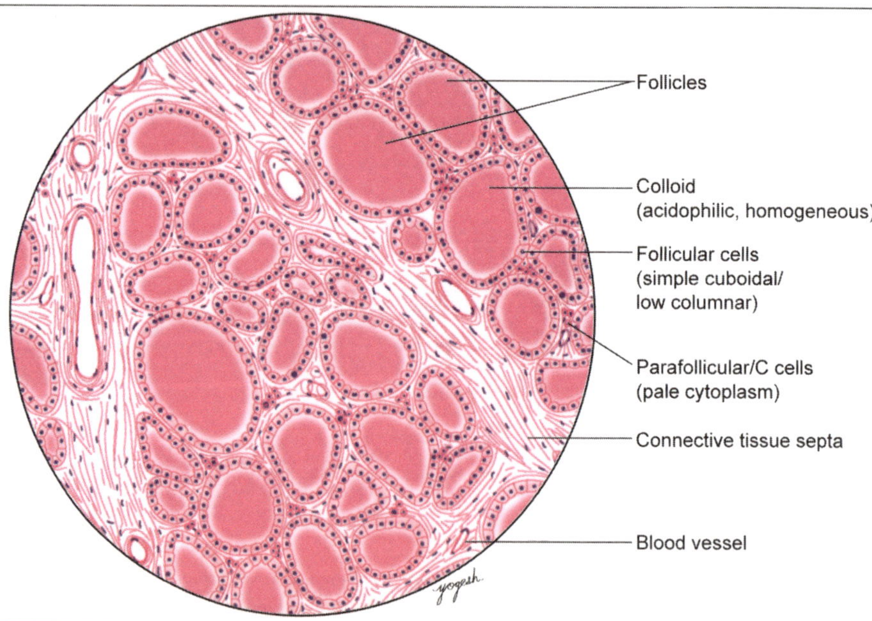


Thyroid gland is consists of follicles lined by simple cuboidal epithelium (squamous to low columnar) with rounded nuclei.
Lumen of follicle contains pink homogeneous colloid material that consists of thyroglobulin.
Few parafollicular/C-cells are present in relation to follicles (secrete calcitonin).
In between follicles, rich vascular connective tissue is present.

*Space for Notes* ____________________________

## Plate 85: **Parathyroid Gland**

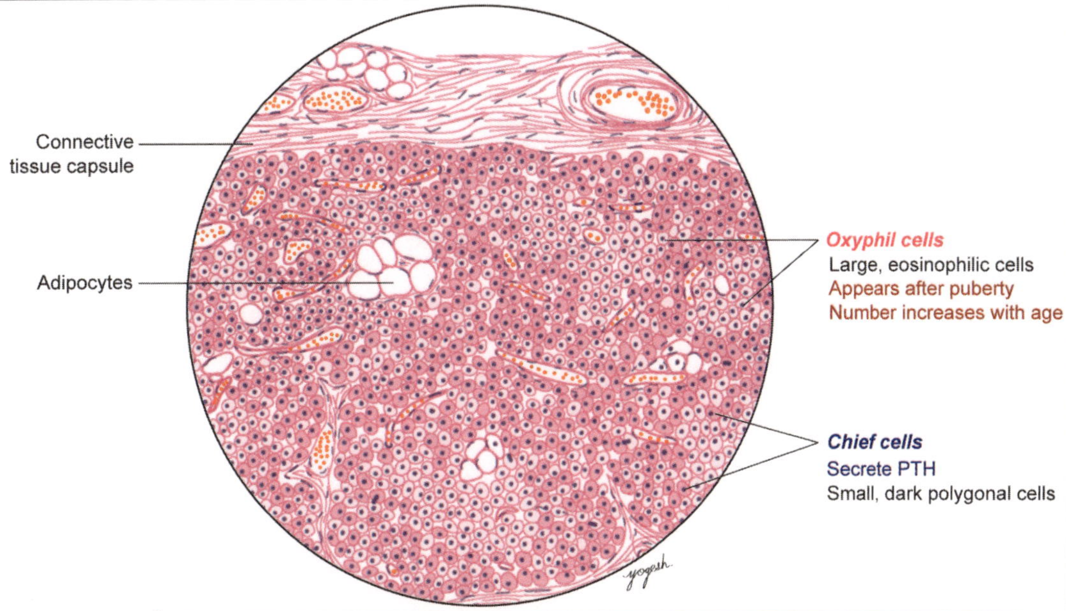


Parathyroid gland shows cords or sheets of cells separated by numerous capillaries.
It shows two types of cells:
Chief cells: more in number, small in size, and consist of a spherical nucleus with small amount of cytoplasm (secrete PTH).
Oxyphil (eosinophilic) cells: less in number, larger in size, small intense-staining nucleus, eosinophilic cytoplasm (no secretion).

## Plate 86: **Cerebrum**

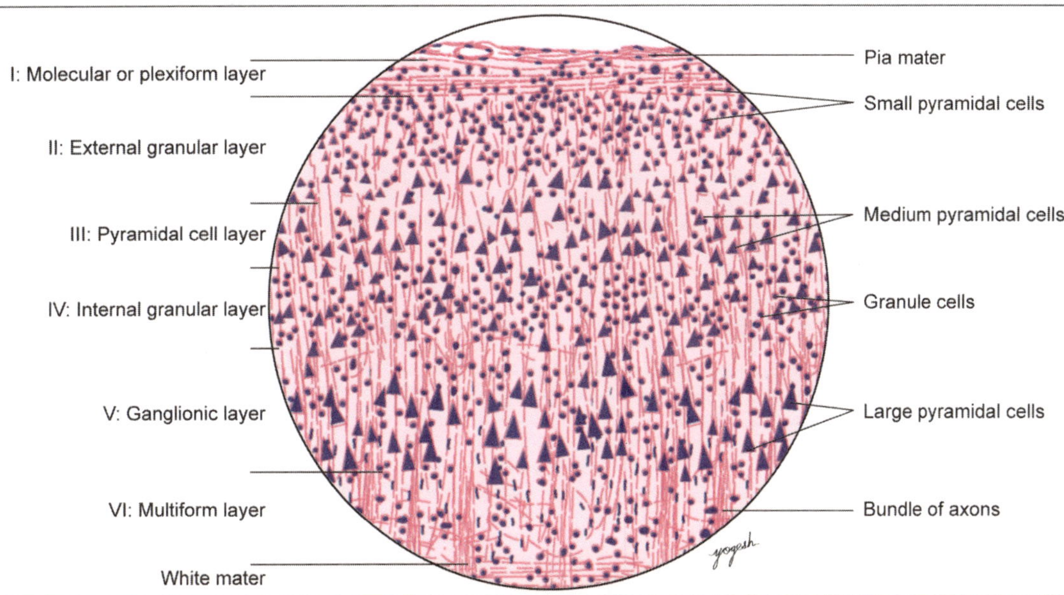


Cerebrum consists of outer grey matter (6 layered) and inner white matter. Layers of cerebral cortex are as follows:

I. Outermost molecular (plexiform) layer consists mainly nerve fibers and few horizontal cells of Cajal.
II. External granular layer consists of small pyramidal cells and few stellate/granule cells.
III. External pyramidal layer consists of medium pyramidal cells, few stellate cells.
IV. Internal granular layer consists of numerous small granulae/stellate cells. It has horizontal fibers – external band of Baillarger.
V. Internal pyramidal layer consists of large pyramidal cells of Betz and horizontal fibers that form internal band of Baillarger.
VI. Multiform layer has spindle-shaped fusiform cells, few stellate cells, and Martinotti cells.

White matter consists of consists of small round nuclei of neuroglial cells and numerous nerve cell processes.

*Space for Notes* ____________

## Plate 87: Cerebellum

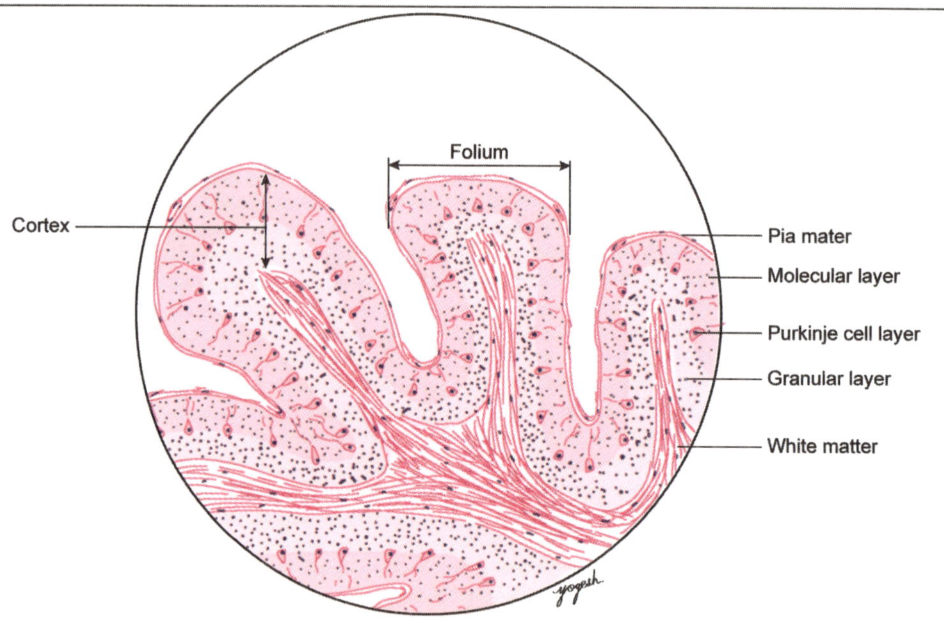


Cerebellum has outer cortex (gray matter) and inner white matter.
Gray matter has three layers:
1. Molecular layer is lighter on H&E staining. It has numerous nerve fibers, stellate cells, basket cells, and neuroglia.
2. Purkinje cell layer consists of a single row of flask shaped Purkinje cells.
3. Granular layer is dark on H&E staining. It has numerous small granule cells and larger Golgi cells.

White matter is composed of fibers and neuroglial cells.

## Plate 88: Spinal Cord (H&E Staining)

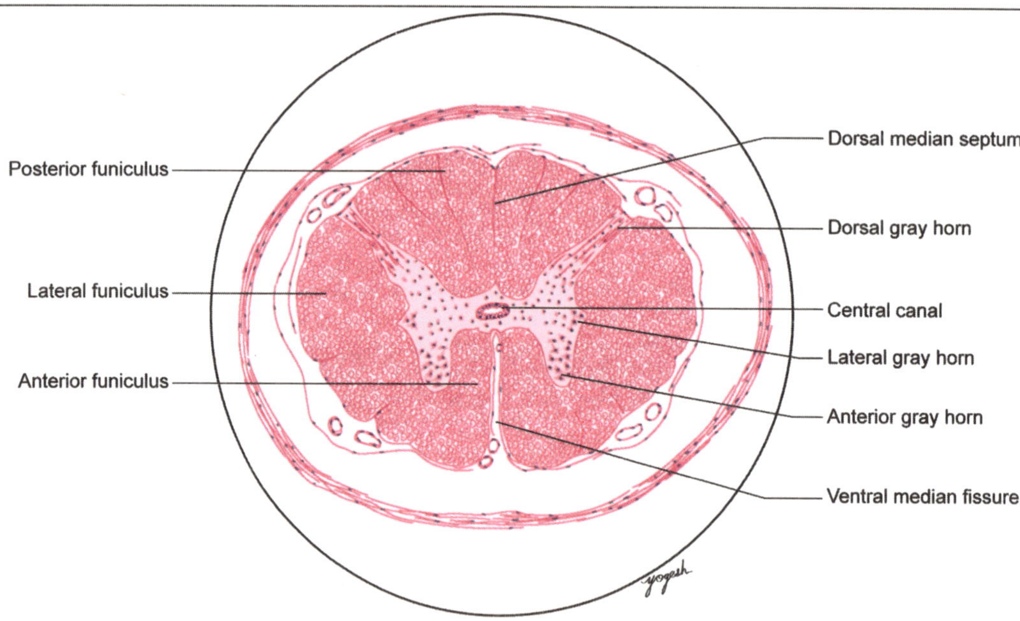


Spinal cord consists of inner gray matter, outer white matter, and central ependyma-lined central canal.
Gray matter has: Anterior horn—shows large multipolar anterior horn cells; Posterior horn—shows small neurons
White matter consists of posterior, lateral, and anterior white columns. These columns have myelinated axons that are surrounded by neuroglial cells.

*Space for Notes* ______________________________

## Plate 89: Spinal Cord at Different Levels

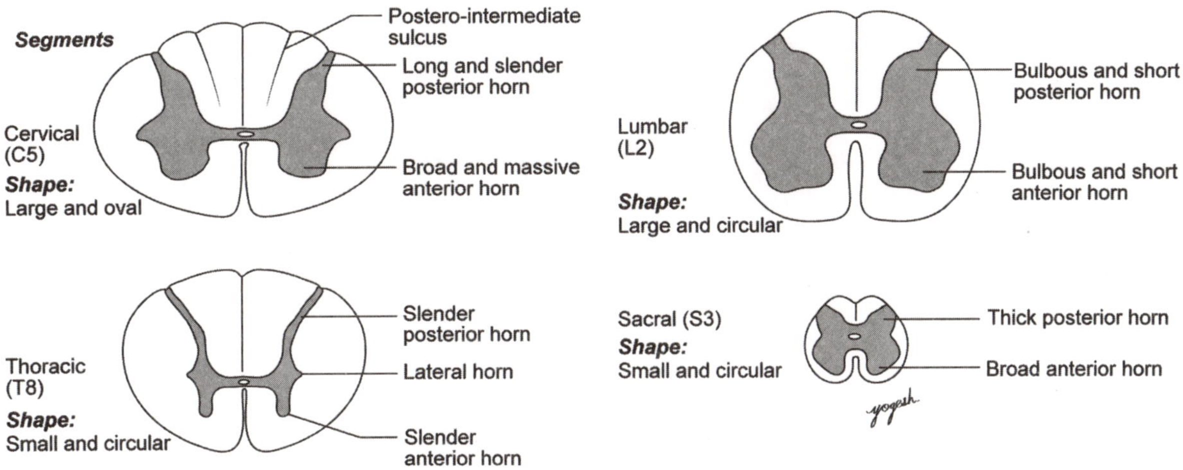


## Plate 90: Cornea

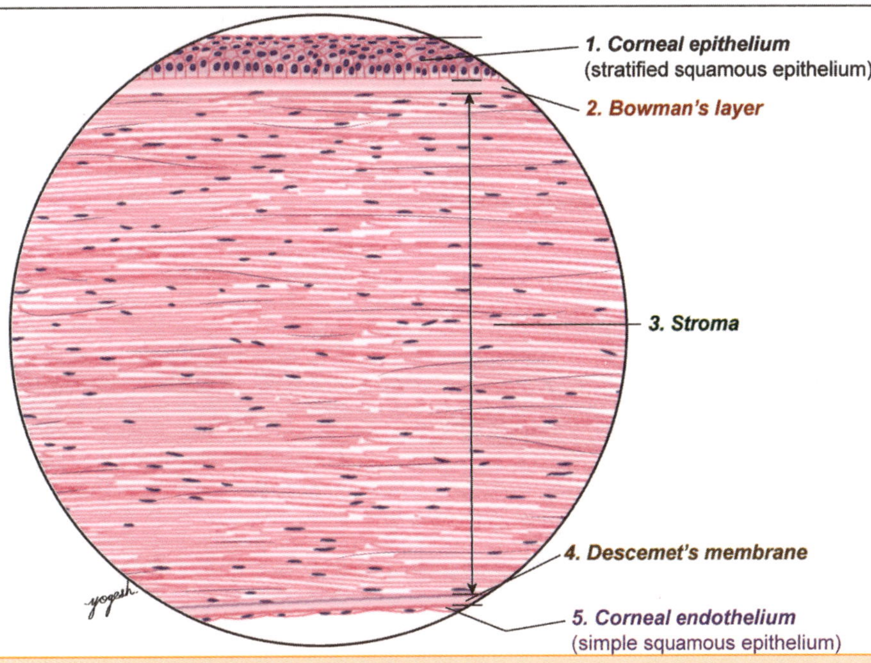


Cornea has five layers:

1. Corneal epithelium consists of nonkeratinized stratified squamous epithelium.
2. Bowman's membrane/anterior limiting lamina is thickened basal lamina of corneal epithelium.
3. Corneal stroma consists of layers of collagen fibrils and few fibroblasts.
4. Descemet's membrane/posterior limiting lamina is the thickened basal lamina of corneal endothelium.
5. Posterior endothelium consists of simple squamous (low cuboidal) epithelium.

*Space for Notes* ______

## Plate 91: **Retina**

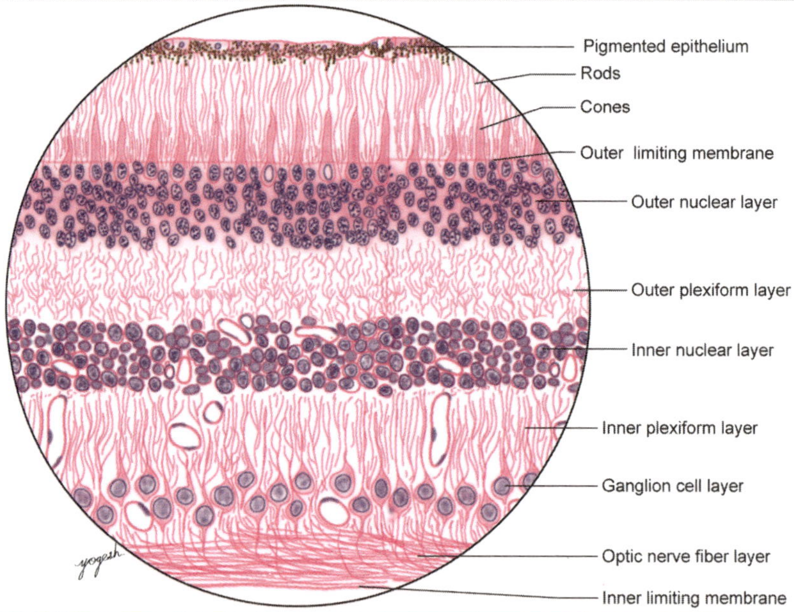


Layers of retina from outside inward:
1. Retinal pigment epithelium: Outermost layer—single layer of cuboidal cells containing melanin.
2. Layer of rods and cones. 3. Outer limiting membrane 4. Outer nuclear layer—consists of nuclei of rods and cones.
5. Outer plexiform layer. 6. Inner nuclear layer
7. Inner plexiform layer 8. Ganglion cell layer—contains nuclei of ganglion cells.
9. Layer of optic nerve fibers 10. Inner limiting membrane

## Plate 92: **Optic Nerve — Transverse Section**

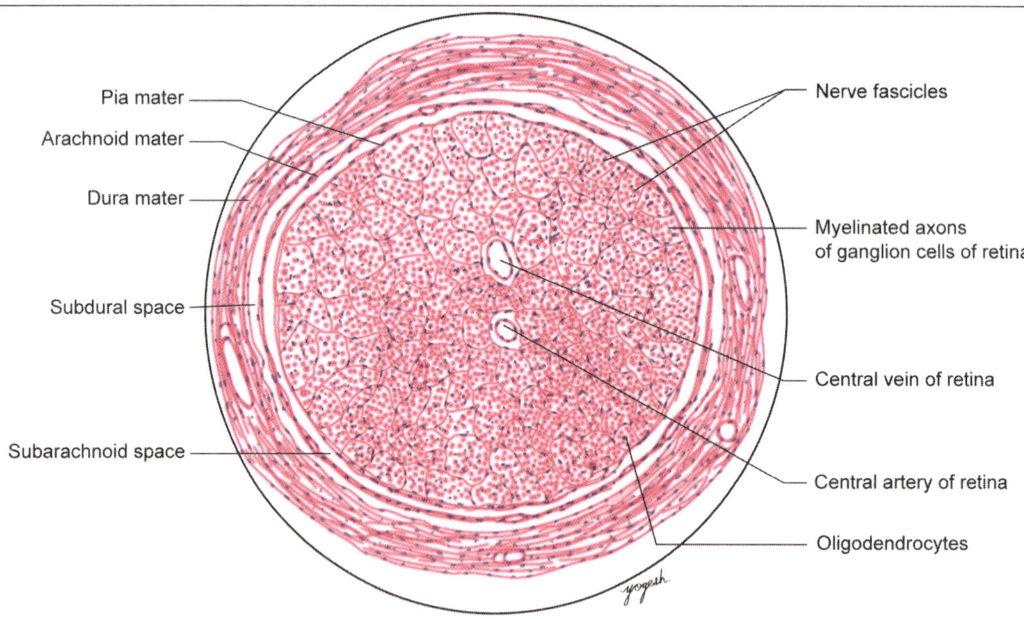


Optic nerve is covered by three sheaths: Outermost dura mater, middle arachnoid mater, and innermost pia mater.
From pia mater, septa arise that divide optic nerve into number of fascicles.
Each fascicle consists of myelinated axons of ganglion cells of retina. Each axon is surrounded by myelin.
In the center of optic nerve, central artery and vein of retina are present.

*Space for Notes* __________

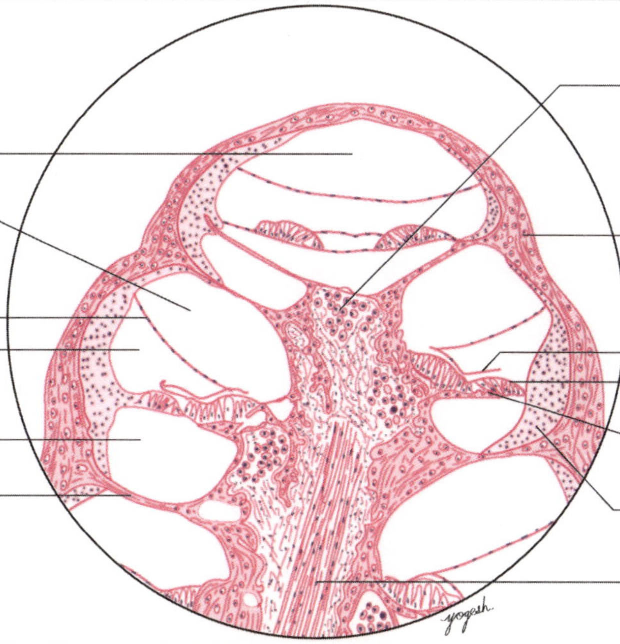


Bony cochlear canal is divided into scala vestibuli above and scala tympani below and they are filled with perilymph.
Scala media lies between scala vestibuli and scala tympani and is filled with endolymph.
Basilar membrane is a fibrous sheet, and it supports the organ of Corti which is innervated by spiral ganglion.
Vestibular/Reissner's membrane separates scala media from scala vestibuli.
Stria vascularis is highly vascular zone in the lateral wall of cochlear duct.

*Space for Notes*